PRACTICAL PATHOLOGY FOR THE MASSAGE THERAPIST

Su Fox

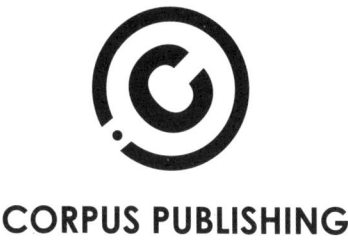

CORPUS PUBLISHING

© Corpus Publishing Limited 2005

Corpus Publishing Limited
PO Box 8, Lydney, Gloucestershire, GL15 6YD, United Kingdom.

Disclaimer
This publication is intended as an informational guide. The techniques described are a supplement to, and not a substitute for, professional tuition. While the information herein is supplied in good faith, no responsibility is taken either by the publisher or by the author for any damage, injury or loss, however caused, which may arise from the use of the information provided.

British Library Cataloguing in Publication Data
A CIP record for this book is available from the British Library
ISBN 1 903333 19 9

Printed and bound in Great Britain by Cambrian Printers

Contents

	Introduction	5
1.	Liaising with doctors and other health professionals	9
2.	Massage and medication	16
3.	Common medical procedures	27
4.	Indications and contraindications	32
5.	Disease	35
6.	Musculoskeletal disorders	40
7.	Skin disorders	58
8.	Cardiovascular disorders	71
9.	Respiratory disorders	83
10.	Pain and nociception	91
11.	Nervous system disorders	93
12.	Massage for the physically vulnerable	106
13.	Sensory disorders	109
14.	Communication and cognitive disorders	112
15.	Emotional vulnerability	117
16.	Immune disorders	123
17.	Endocrine disorders	130
18.	Digestive disorders	134
19.	Female reproductive processes	142
20.	Reproductive system disorders	144
21.	Sexually transmitted diseases	147
22.	Massage and sexuality	149
23.	Urinary system disorders	151
	References	155
	Index	157

Acknowledgements

Material in this book is taken in part from Fox & Pritchard's *Anatomy, Physiology and Pathology for the Massage Therapist*.

Much of the material in this book was first published as articles in *Massage World* magazine between 2003 and 2004.

Thanks to Wendy Kavanagh, editor of *Massage World*, for suggesting I write the articles in the first place.

To Rik Fox, consultant anaesthetist at the Royal National Orthopaedic Hospital, for helping to clarify some of the cardiovascular conditions, and for information on spinal injuries, massage and medication.

To Leonard Easton, former gynacologist at the Royal London Hospital, for commenting on the section on the reproductive systems.

To Darien Pritchard, Richard Leadbeater, Anja Saunders, Sally Morris and David Le May for general helpful comments.

To Ceris Fender, Jan Elson and Andrew Ravensdale for their help with the sections on working with people with disabilities.

To Andrew Kerr, former massage therapist at London Lighthouse, for his help with the section on HIV/AIDS.

To Andy Fagg, massage specialist at the Bristol Cancer Help Centre, for comments on massage and cancer.

To all the people I've taught or massaged over the years from whom I've learnt more about medical conditions than I have ever learnt from a book.

And to Gina Barker for her support, patience and encouragement.

Introduction

Why do we need to know about pathology?

Pathology is the branch of medicine that studies the things that go wrong with the tissues and workings of the body. The word 'pathological' does have vaguely sinister associations, but it is worth considering that all of us have some sort of pathology.

One dictionary definition of 'pathology' is: 'any variant or deviation from the norm'. According to this definition, short sight, skin sensitivity to bergamot oil, athlete's foot or an allergy to tomatoes are all pathological. Spend a moment remembering all the ailments, childhood illnesses, accidents or operations you've had during your lifetime. That's your personal history of pathology.

Once upon a time, massage was a luxury or a slightly dubious activity associated with massage parlours. Thankfully, with continued professionalism and public education, the association between massage and sex is fading, and many more people are turning to massage for reasons of health and well-being. As many as one in three people have tried some sort of complementary therapy.

There are various reasons for this increased interest, one being that complementary therapists are often able to offer more individual attention, time and care than practitioners working in the public health sector. Another reason is that many people try complementary therapy because they are dissatisfied with the treatment they've received from their doctor or hospital. So, these days, a person booking a massage treatment may well be suffering from some sort of medical condition, and it is incumbent on the therapist to have a basic understanding of pathology so that he or she can make informed decisions about how to massage safely and effectively.

There are, of course, frameworks other than the traditional medical model for understanding and helping when things go wrong with the body. Acupuncture, shiatsu, polarity therapy and healing are all examples of energy-based therapies, which, in their different ways, work by unblocking and balancing the flow of energies in and around the body through direct contact with the body. Medicinal complementary therapies, such as naturopathy or homoeopathy, use extracts from plants or minerals to treat the underlying causes of a problem rather than treating the symptoms.

Many complementary therapies have an underlying belief that there is an inherent ability in the body to heal itself, given the right conditions, and it is the job of the therapist to facilitate this self-healing. The therapies that deal with the mind and emotion, such as counselling, psychotherapy, relaxation training and meditation understand that how we think and feel has a role in our physical well-being. The ideal for the holistic massage therapist is, maybe, to be able to hold in mind several frameworks at once – anatomical, energetic, mental and emotional – and for these frameworks to inform his understanding of the story each client tells about her body.

Pathology and massage

However, when it comes to pathology it is important for the massage practitioner to understand the theoretical basis of the medical model, and to be familiar with medical terminology. Just as a solid grounding in anatomy, particularly musculo-skeletal, enables the practitioner to massage more effectively, and an understanding of physiology helps the practitioner to recognise the connection between stress, arousal, relaxation and the functioning of the nervous system, so a basic knowledge of pathology is essential for understanding the rationale behind contraindications, and how to massage safely. It enables us to communicate credibly with medical practitioners, and increases our clients' confidence in us as professionals who know what we are doing. Having said that, we are not medical practitioners and it is not our job to diagnose or to treat medical complaints, unless we are trained in remedial or sports massage and can do this for musculo-skeletal problems. We don't need to know a lot about medical conditions either, just enough to make a good treatment decision.

With a knowledge of pathology, the practitioner can make sense of medical information from the client in terms of which body systems are involved and the likely effects on the relevant body tissues and areas. Further questioning about the condition (such as what medication is being taken, and how the condition affects that particular person) can then help the practitioner decide how to adapt the session for that client's needs. This includes practical issues, such as the kinds of supports needed, the temperature of the room, the use of oil or cream, whether to remove clothes or not, or whether to lie down or not. Knowledge of pathology can inform decisions about the treatment itself: where to focus, where to be careful, where to avoid, and the depth, speed and rhythm of strokes. Having an understanding of the client's condition also helps to ascertain 'safety' information. For example, if the client is severely asthmatic, has she got her ventilator with her?

Chapter 1

Liaising with doctors and other health professionals

The aim of this book is to provide information about common medical conditions, underlying causes, signs and symptoms, and indications and contraindications for massage, to help you make good choices about how to adapt your skills safely for any client, and to have the confidence to work with clients who are not well and healthy. For a more comprehensive list of pathological conditions, it is a good idea to have a simple medical dictionary, access to a good website, and a copy of the *British National Formulary* for information about medication.

When treating people who are currently receiving medical treatment it is also sensible and responsible to liaise with the client's doctor or consultant, just as it is sensible to liaise with other complementary therapists your client may be seeing. The question is how to know when to liaise and when not to. If you were to send away every client who is at all unwell until a doctor's letter of consent to massage is provided, you would lose a lot of clients and create considerable frustration and disappointment, and you might wait forever for the expected letter. Some clients don't want to tell their doctors that they are receiving complementary therapy. Some doctors may be sceptical about the benefits of massage, and all are extremely busy people.

Guidelines within the massage profession vary a lot, and, as yet, there are no clear recommendations about medical liaison. The phrase 'get the doctor's permission before you massage' is often used. The trouble with this suggestion is that many doctors are unfamiliar with the effects of massage therapy, or different styles of massage, and are not in a position to make a professional decision. And there is something about 'asking permission' that endorses the idea that we massage therapists don't know what we are doing, don't feel as important as doctors, and don't expect to be taken seriously. The idea of informing or consulting with medical practitioners (and other complementary therapists) about our practice, or requesting advice about the advisability of massage, puts us in a position where we take ourselves seriously and expect to be taken seriously by other professions.

Reasons for liaising

1. Courtesy
2. To foster good relations between professions
3. To work as a team for the client's best interests
4. For insurance purposes
5. To request information

If Doris Smith has a complicated medical history, or a

chronic condition, or is taking a number of medications, she already has an on-going and possibly long-standing relationship with a health professional and it is only courteous to inform that person that Doris has decided to consult you as well. Communicating in a responsible manner helps to build good relationships between the massage and medical professions. This also applies to other complementary therapists. If, for example, Asad Kahn has been seeing a chiropractor for low back pain, informing the other practitioner that he is also coming to you for massage enables you all to schedule the appointments, and perhaps modify treatments, so that Mr Kahn gets the best possible care for his back problem.

Liaison with the medical profession is also important for insurance purposes. Although none of the main British insurance companies exclude any medical conditions from massage treatment, all recommend that a full medical history is taken, including treatments and medications, and that a doctor's consent is obtained. Were a client to take a massage therapist to court, claiming that treatment had aggravated a medical condition, the counter claim could be argued more effectively if there had been medical contact. In this respect, liaison is a safeguard for the therapist.

Another possible reason for liaising with a doctor or consultant is to ask for specific advice. If, for example, the vague muscular aches and pains that Anna White gave as her main reason for having massage haven't improved after a few sessions, and you know that she takes an anti-depressant, and you also know that a side effect of some antidepressants is muscular aches and pains, you may decide to write to her doctor for an opinion on the matter. Or if someone with a terminal condition requests massage privately, you may choose to contact his doctor to discuss how you can best be part of his palliative care team.

How to liaise

There are different ways to consider liaising. Bearing in mind that all information a client gives you is confidential, if you decide to communicate with another practitioner you must discuss this with the client, giving clear reasons for your decision, and you must have your client's consent. You could then ask the client to inform her doctor verbally, at her next appointment, that she has started to have massage treatment. This is a very informal approach. The problems with it are that you have no evidence, apart from the client's word, about the doctor's response and no written evidence, in case of a malpractice claim. Another is to write to the doctor with the information that you are currently seeing her patient for massage, and to request that if she has any observations or reservations, to let you know. You could have a standard letter for such purposes. Keep a copy on file and a copy of any responses. A third approach is to write a more detailed letter requesting information about the advisability of massage from the doctor. If, for example, a client has had a stroke, you might want the go ahead from his doctor about when it is safe for him to receive massage.

If a client refuses permission to liaise, you have two choices. If you have serious doubts, either about the advisability of massage with a particular medical condition, or about your own experience and competence to massage safely, then don't. Explain your reservations and possibly refer to another practitioner.

The other choice is to ask the client to sign a medical disclaimer, to the effect that he refused permission to consult with his doctor and takes full responsibility for his medical condition and any changes that arise as a result of having massage.

However, as the professional, you still have total responsibility for the treatment, including anything detrimental that could happen, and a written disclaimer holds no legal weight were a malpractice case to be brought by the client.

When to liaise

How to decide when to inform, when to ask about the advisability of massage, and when not to bother? Throughout the book there are recommendations for specific conditions about consultation with the medical profession. The following lists are suggestions only and are not intended as absolute criteria. Use your commonsense in each individual case, use the guidelines in this book, or ask your professional organisation or training college, or an experienced colleague about medical liaison and, of course, ask for the client's consent.

Don't bother…

- Mild to moderate strains and sprains, and cramp.

- Common complaints for which the client is not receiving medical treatment, including upper respiratory infections, such as colds, coughs, sinusitis, common allergies, such as hay fever, jet lag, constipation/diarrhoea (unless part of an underlying condition).
- Localised skin conditions, unless they are severe or undiagnosed.
- Visual and hearing impairment.
- Conditions that have resolved or are in remission, and there is no ongoing medical treatment.
- Common menstrual or menopausal symptoms.
- Pregnancy, unless there is a history of miscarriage.

Inform the doctor

- Unhealed fractures, all types of arthritis and osteoporosis.
- RSIs, muscular dystrophy, fibromyalgia.
- Severe or widespread skin disorders for which the client is receiving medical treatment.
- Severe respiratory conditions, such as emphysema, chronic bronchitis and pneumonia.
- Most nervous system disorders affecting motor and/or sensory function if the client has ongoing medical treatment.
- Clients who are emotionally vulnerable and taking medication – but be sensitive to the client's wishes.
- Cancer, if in remission.
- Diabetes, thyroid and other endocrine disorders.
- Disorders of the large intestine, such as Crohn's disease, or irritable bowel syndrome (IBS).
- Gall and kidney stones.

Ask the doctor about the advisability of massage

- Recent major surgery.
- Cancer, if in treatment.
- HIV/AIDS, if seriously unwell.
- Most cardiovascular conditions.
- Conditions that are infectious for a certain period during the acute phase, such as pulmonary TB.
- Hepatitis and cirrhosis.

Chapter 2
Massage and medication

Medication is prescribed because something has gone wrong with the body. Drugs can relieve pain (the analgesics), fight bacterial infection (antibiotics), alter the consistency of the blood, the diameter of blood vessels or airways, change hormone levels, disperse water retention, affect mood and have many other uses. Drugs are designed and prescribed to alter the physiology of the body. Since massage may also alter the physiology of the body, there is the possibility that someone on prescribed drugs may respond to a massage treatment in an unpredictable way. For example, a client with a sore shoulder may have rubbed ibuprofen, a common analgesic for muscular pain, on the area. Because ibuprofen reduces the ability of the blood to clot, a deep tissue massage may cause bruising and discomfort rather than relief.

Another factor of relevance to massage therapists is that the side effects of some medication are identical to common ailments. For example, a common side effect of antidepressants is joint and muscle pain. A person taking an antidepressant who comes for massage may not experience any long-term improvement in these symptoms because they are drug-induced.

It is important to take a full drug history as part of the initial case history so that you can alter your treatment accordingly. Many people don't know the full name of their medication but will tell you it's for their water/blood pressure/nerves. If the client is unsure, ask him to write the name down or bring his pills or medicine at the next visit.

The *British National Formulary* (BNF) is a book compiled by the British Medical Association and The Royal Pharmaceutical Society, which lists all current medications on the market, together with their uses, contraindications and side effects. This guide is updated every year, so it is worth asking your local surgery or health-care centre if you could have a back copy before it gets thrown out.

When reading about side effects, bear in mind that, even if only one person has reported a particular symptom as a result of taking the drug, it has to go in the list of side effects! In the BNF you will find information about your client's medication that may help inform your treatment decisions. If in doubt, consult with the client's doctor about the advisability of massage.

ROUTE OF ADMINISTRATION

It is also important to ask how the medication is taken into the body, since this can have consequences for the massage treatment. Drugs that are taken orally and absorbed into the bloodstream, as well as drops into the eyes or ears, sprays into the nose or throat, pessaries and suppositories, do not interact directly with a massage treatment and the only consideration might be the timing of a treatment in relation to release of the drug into the system. For this information, consult the client's doctor.

Topical preparations

Topical preparations are ones that are applied on to the skin. These include creams, ointments or gels for skin conditions, such as Betnovate, those for relief of muscular aches and pains, such as ibuprofen, and those for disorders of other systems, which can be absorbed into the blood through the skin. This last group includes patches for HRT administration. Patches provide slow release of the drug involved and are increasingly common.

Cautions for massage

Never wipe off a topical preparation that has just been applied – treat as a local contraindication. Avoid an area of several inches around a patch. Disturbing a patch carries a risk of therapist exposure to the medication.

Injection

There are various ways that drugs given by injection are introduced into the body. The most common routes are subcutaneous (just under the skin), intramuscular (directly into muscle), intra-articular (directly into a joint), and intravenous (directly into a vein). Most are quick release, which means that the medication disperses from the site within a few hours, but some are slow release and active for much longer. The hormone therapy prescribed for prostate cancer lasts up to six weeks, and there is a contraceptive given by injection that lasts several months.

Cautions for massage

If the injection is quick release and not part of an ongoing series of injections, for example travel vaccinations, treat the site as a local contraindication for 24 hours unless inflammation is still present. If the injection is slow release, always treat the site as a local contraindication. Intramuscular injections often cause inflammation and tenderness – treat the site as a local contraindication until the symptoms have resolved. Old intramuscular sites that have been used repeatedly become fibrous, and techniques for scar tissue could be used carefully.

Implants

Implants are mechanical aids attached to the body either to drain fluids, like a urine catheter, or to administer drugs. Implants are rare, and usually a person with an implant would be in hospital or in a care home. An exception to this is the Hickman line, a little device that is embedded in the chest, and used to administer drugs for HIV/AIDS or cancer.

Cautions for massage

A person with a Hickman line knows how to handle it. Negotiate about use of supports for comfort when he is lying on his front. Treat the whole chest area as a local contraindication and avoid getting oil on the device.

Analgesics (painkillers)

There are four types of painkillers that act on the body in different ways and are used for different kinds of medical conditions. They can be taken orally, by injection or used as creams or gels for local application.

1. Non-steroid anti-inflammatory drugs (NSAIDs) work by preventing the production of certain chemicals from damaged cells. These chemicals contribute to pain and inflammation. NSAIDs help to reduce inflammation and they also thin the blood. They are used in inflammatory conditions like rheumatoid arthritis, for mild to moderate pain from injury, muscular complaints, osteoarthritis, and some cardiovascular disorders. The most common one is ibuprofen (Nurofen), available over the counter, and Voltarol, which is only available on prescription.

Cautions for massage

NSAIDs alter the clotting ability of the blood. A person taking an oral NSAID or using a cream locally may bruise more easily. Deep tissue work is inadvisable.

All analgesics alter sensory perception and reduce the client's ability to give accurate feedback about discomfort or pain. Remember this when using joint stretches or manipulations.

2. Corticosteroid anti-inflammatory drugs act in the same way as the corticosteroids produced naturally by the adrenal glands. They have an anti-inflammatory effect, alter metabolism of glucose, and depress immune-system functioning. They are very widely prescribed for a range of conditions, including auto-immune diseases, allergic conditions, and chronic skin conditions like psoriasis. They tend to be used for more severe or chronic conditions than the NSAIDs.

Examples of corticosteroids include Cortisone, a cream used to treat muscular inflammation and repetitive strain injuries, and Becatide, an asthma medication. Prednisolone is a corticosteroid often used for long-term connective tissue disorders, including rheumatoid arthritis.

Cautions for massage

Corticosteroids suppress normal immune system functioning, which means that someone taking them is more susceptible to infection. Take extra precautions with hygiene and do not treat if you have an infection yourself.

Long-term use of corticosteroids results in thin skin. Use gentle massage only. If a cream is used, avoid the affected area.

Long-term high doses of corticosteroids affect the resilience of all the muscles and connective tissues, making them fragile, easier to damage and less well able to heal. Avoid deep tissue, friction, percussion techniques and heavy pressure on muscles, bones or joints.

3. Opiates, or narcotic analgesics, act like the body's own opiate neurochemicals, which are the ones that produce positive feelings. The 'endorphin high' described by long-distance runners is caused by the release of the opiate called endorphin.

These drugs are potentially addictive, and are only available on prescription. Co-proxamol is a painkiller that contains an opiate derivative. Methadone, which is used in drug rehabilitation programmes, and morphine, which is used in terminal illness, are both strong opiates. These drugs are also used for severe pain from fractures, major surgery or injury, and for chronic pain syndromes. They are only available on prescription.

Cautions for massage

The opiates can cause dizziness, sleepiness or light-headed feelings. Take care at the end of the treatment to get the client off the table safely, and ensure that she is steady enough when she leaves.

Like the other analgesics, sensory feedback from the body is affected and the client will not be able to give accurate feedback. Remember this when using joint stretches or manipulations.

4. Muscle relaxants are used to reduce spasticity or muscle spasm in skeletal muscle. Some act on the central, and some on the peripheral, nervous system. Although they act on the motor nerves or directly on muscle fibres, sensory input may also be impaired.

Cautions for massage

The muscles tend to feel flaccid and unresponsive. Observe the recommendations for massage with clients with muscle conditions. Avoid over stretching.

Mood-altering medications

Antidepressant drugs work by altering the balance of neurotransmitters relating to mood and are used to treat depression, obsessional disorders and severe pain from cancer. There are two sorts: the tricyclic antidepressants and the serotonin reuptake inhibitors (SSRIs). Prozac and Seroxat are SSRIs.

Mild tranquillisers are given to reduce anxiety, for insomnia and as muscle relaxants. They suppress central nervous system functioning. An examples is diazepam (valium).

Anti-psychotic drugs are used to treat symptoms of delusion and hallucination, and severe thought disturbance. Examples are Largactyl and Stelazine.

Cautions for massage

A person taking a mood-altering medication is likely to be emotionally vulnerable. Observe the recommendations for massage in Chapter 15. On a physiological level, all these drugs have side effects, different for each type, and you may need to check whether the client's symptoms are drug-related. As mentioned previously, joint and muscle pain are common side effects, and, as such, will not be relieved by massage.

These drugs can cause dizziness, sleepiness or light-headed feelings. Take care at the end of the treatment to get the client off the table safely, and ensure that he is steady enough when he leaves.

Fatigue is another common experience. Depending on the client's general vitality, you may need to shorten the treatment time. General relaxation massage is probably the best option.

Cardiovascular medications

Cardiovascular disorders are complex and so are the medications to treat them. A person with a cardiovascular complaint may well be taking more than one kind. Try to find out exactly what and look up the side effects to ascertain which of the reported symptoms might be due to the drugs. Always liaise with the client's doctor about the advisability of massage.

Beta blockers are drugs that slow down heart rate. They are used for angina and high blood pressure and sometimes for anxiety.

Vasodilators are various types of drugs that increase the diameter of blood vessels, to improve blood flow.

Anticoagulants are prescribed for people with a history of DVT or clots, and literally 'thin the blood'.

Diuretics is the general name for drugs that stimulate urination, reduce blood volume and increase the release of water from the body. They are used for high blood pressure and other disorders, such as oedema brought about by heart failure.

Cautions for massage

Breathing difficulties may occur. Consider treating the client sitting up, and keep drinking water handy.

Some vasodilators increase the risk of a DVT. If the client reports swollen, tired legs and feet, treat as a total contraindication and refer them to their doctor.

People on anticoagulants bleed more easily, so care should be taken to avoid heavy pressure during treatment. Help the client on and off the couch.

The need to urinate frequently and urgently is common with people taking diuretics. Ask if the client wants to use the toilet before the treatment, and be prepared to interrupt the massage if necessary.

Medications for respiratory disorders

Antihistamines counteract the effect of histamine, a substance produced by the body as part of the allergic response. They are used not only for respiratory problems but all kinds of allergic reactions. Drowsiness is a well-known side effect.

Bronchodilators act by dilating the bronchioles. Salbutamol and Ventolin are the most widely used bronchodilators. Asthmatics and other people with chronic breathing difficulties often use inhalers containing these drugs.

Decongestants work by suppressing the production of mucous in the nasal passages.

Cautions for massage

Many medications for respiratory disorders cause dryness of the mouth, nasal cavity and trachea, which in turn causes irritation and coughing. Have drinking water available for the client.

A common side effect is drowsiness or light-headedness. Take care at the end of the treatment to get the client off the table safely.

Antibiotics

The first antibiotic discovered was penicillin. The most common one today is amoxycillin. Antibiotics are taken orally to treat a number of bacterial infections. Over the years many bacteria have developed strains that are resistant to antibiotics.

Cautions for massage

The reason for the person taking an antibiotic needs to be taken into account when planning the massage treatment, but antibiotics do not alter physiology in a way that is affected by massage.

Chapter 3
Common medical procedures

A basic knowledge of common medical procedures can be helpful for the massage practitioner. It helps to understand what a client is talking about when he says he's had an MRI scan, for example, and may help to make sense of the results in a way that is useful to planning treatment.

X-rays

This procedure projects minute amounts of radiation into the body, and a black-and-white image is produced. X-rays show bones, lungs and heart clearly, but are less accurate for other tissues. The person being X-rayed stands, sits or lies in front of the X-ray machine for a short time.

Barium X-rays

If barium salts are introduced into the digestive tract, these softer tissues also show up well on X-rays. There are different methods for different parts of the tract. A barium swallow is a drink that shows up in the oesophagus and top of the stomach, a barium meal is similar but the patient has to lie down and wait for the drink to reach the stomach and duodenum, and a barium enema shows up problems in the colon. The patient has to fast or follow a special diet a few days before a barium X-ray. These procedures may be uncomfortable but are not generally painful.

Bone scans

Bone scans are used to check bones for fractures or tumours, and show unusual lumps or distortions. A small amount of a radioactive material that concentrates around inflammation in bones is injected into a vein. Painless except for the initial injection, a bone scan can take several hours.

Bone-density scan (DEXA scan)

Similar to having an X-ray, except that areas focused on are the hip and lumbar vertebra, this kind of scan determines the relative density of a portion of bone, and compares it to normal density for a person of that age. This is used for diagnosing osteoporosis.

CT scan

To have a CT scan, the patient lies down and his body is inserted slowly into a short tunnel. This technique takes lots of X-rays of a particular part of the body, from different angles, and puts them into a computer. Images of thin slices of body, showing all tissues and abnormalities, are produced.

MRI scan

To have an MRI, the patient lies down and his body is inserted slowly into a large metal cylinder, which scans in great detail. It shows different body tissues in different colours. The method involves magnetism not radiation.

CT and MRI procedures are painless but time-consuming. An MRI scan can be difficult for someone who feels claustrophobic.

Ultrasound scanning

Ultrasound is a high-frequency sound wave that is directed at tissues, and the waves that are reflected back are monitored for information about that tissue.

Ultrasound machines are portable and are moved over the relevant area of the patient's body. Ultrasound is also used by physiotherapists to break up scar tissue in muscles and connective tissue, and to promote healing.

Mammogram

Mammograms screen for the presence of breast cancer and are recommended for all women over 50. The breasts are placed between two X-ray plates, a quick procedure that may be uncomfortable but doesn't hurt.

Endoscopy

Endoscopy is the investigation of the internal tissues using a flexible thin telescope with fibre optics at the end. The instrument can be passed down the oesophagus to look at the stomach (gastroscopy), or into the rectum (colonoscopy). These two procedures are done under local anaesthetic or sedation. The others are done under general anaesthetic and sometimes surgical interventions, like the removal of damaged tissue, are performed at the same time. Laparoscopy is the investigation of the abdomen or pelvis through a small incision in the abdominal wall, bronchoscopy of the lungs and thoracic cavity and arthroscopy of the joints.

CARDIOVASCULAR TESTS

ECG (electrocardiogram)

An ECG tests heart rate and rhythm. Electrodes are attached to the patient's arm and chest, usually sitting down, and his heart rate is recorded on a moving strip of paper. An exercise ECG is a record of heart rate during exercise on a treadmill.

Angiogram/arteriogram

These tests involve introducing a dye into the arteries and using X-ray to determine the state of the vessels. In the case of an angiogram, a tube carrying the dye is inserted into a vein at the top of the leg and guided to the heart, where the surrounding arteries are investigated.

Blood test

This involves taking a sample of blood from a vein in the

arm. Numerous tests to analyse the contents of the blood can then be carried out, including blood group, blood cell counts, hormone levels, clotting ability, haemoglobin levels, urea and uric acid levels, thyroid function and the presence of viruses, bacteria and antibodies. A doctor may ask for a blood test for a specific purpose, or a full blood count can be carried out, which is a detailed analysis of all possible variables.

ESR (erythrocyte sedimentation rate)

ESR is a blood test that is useful for identifying the presence of an inflammatory disease, such as arthritis, some cancers, and connective tissue disorders.

EEG (electroencephalogram)

This is similar to an ECG, but measures the electrical activity of the brain. Electrodes are attached to the scalp and the results recorded on moving paper. It is painless.

Chapter 4
Indications and contraindications

These are terms from medical practice and refer to whether a particular treatment is 'indicated', meaning 'good for' a particular condition, or harmful (or may cause harmful side effects), in which case it is contra (against) indicated.

Surgery is the indicated treatment for appendicitis, but not for bronchitis. Many medications are contraindicated in pregnancy, because of possible harm to the foetus. Massage could be said to be 'indicated' for muscular tension and stiffness, for stress and associated conditions, and for temporary pain relief.

But what about contraindications? A list of conditions that are contraindications, conditions that we don't massage, isn't very helpful. We need to be able to think much more flexibly, with different categories of contraindications, and even then, to be able to know when something is a hard-and-fast rule, such as avoiding abdominal massage in the first trimester of pregnancy, and when something is a recommendation and your decision depends on a number of factors, including your own common sense. For example, it is generally not recommended to massage a person with an infectious airborne condition that you could catch yourself. Usually someone with such a condition would be feeling too unwell to have a massage anyway. But supposing a client turns up with a bad cold. What do you do? Send him home or have an extra box of tissues to hand?

Total contraindications

There are very few conditions that are total contraindications, where massage is not recommended at all. These fall into two categories.

There are conditions that are infectious, and could be transmitted to the practitioner, or, in some cases, spread to other parts of the client's body, and there are the potentially life-threatening conditions that carry a high risk of reoccurrence. Both of these total contraindications are to protect the practitioner, the first from catching infection and the second from the accusation that a massage treatment could have triggered another, possibly fatal, episode.

In the weeks immediately following a heart attack or a stroke, there is a high probability of reoccurrence, which fades over time and with medical treatment. Deep vein thrombosis is also a total contraindication in the initial stage before medication dissolves the clot, and the risk of it detaching from the wall of the blood vessel where it has formed, and travelling around the system where it could lodge in the lungs or brain, has been reduced. During these periods, massage is a total contraindication and thereafter given only in consultation with the client's doctor until a safe period has elapsed.

Local contraindications

These are the obvious 'massage is okay but avoid the area' conditions. We all know not to massage over open, weeping or cut skin, and to avoid areas of fungal infection on the skin, such as athlete's foot. We know that inflammation, bruising and recent fractures are also local contraindications, but if we omit these parts of the body in the same way as an open sore on the skin, and massage the rest of the body as normal then we are doing that body a disservice.

Many local contraindications require that we know how to work with them. An area of inflammation, for example, will benefit from massage techniques in adjacent areas that improve the circulation, and increase the supply of food and oxygen to the damaged tissues while removing wastes. This book will help you think about how to work with local contraindications, where appropriate, rather than avoid them.

Chapter 5
Disease

It's helpful, when thinking about pathology and contraindications, to have an understanding of some of the factors that cause or contribute to disease in the physical body. Very often it isn't possible to pinpoint a single cause, particularly if the whole person and his mental and emotional state and current life situation are taken into account. The virus that causes the common cold, for example, is present in the environment all the time, so why don't we all have constantly runny eyes and blocked noses? Because susceptibility to 'catching' a cold depends on the state of our immune system, which, in turn, can be influenced by how worried, stressed or tired we are. But there are several clear categories of disorder, and in our work as massage therapists we are most likely to encounter the following – infection, trauma and degenerative conditions.

Infection

Infection occurs when another living organism attacks the body. The usual routes of entry to the body are through cuts in the skin, inhaled as droplets in the air through the respiratory tract, or consumed in food or drink and absorbed through the digestive tract. Bacteria or viruses cause most infections.

Bacteria are minute organisms, of varying shapes and sizes, with some of the characteristics of a cell. They are found everywhere, in the air, soil, water and on living creatures. Most bacteria are beneficial and only some cause infections. The skin is home to millions of bacteria that destroy harmful organisms.

Viruses are micro-organisms that cannot exist independently. They need to find their way into the live cells of another organism, where they use the food and energy resources of the host cells to multiply and invade neighbouring cells. Unlike bacteria, they are resistant to antibiotics.

Other infective agents are fungi and parasites. Fungi are a simple form of plant, from the same family as mushrooms, toadstools and the mould that grows on unprotected food. Fungi thrive in moist, warm places. Parasites are more complex organisms that attach to, and feed off, the 'host' organism.

The superbugs

MRSA (Methicillin-resistant Staphylococcus aureus) is one of a number of bacteria that have modified over the years to produce strains that are resistant to antibiotics. MRSA is in the news because of the large increase in MRSA infection in hospital patients. These bacteria live on damp, warm tissues, like those in the armpits, nose or groin, and can survive for a short time in similar conditions outside the body. Thirty per cent of the normal, healthy population are hosts to the MRSA bacteria without being aware of it. For some reason, it doesn't like the other 70 per cent when they are healthy.

MRSA only begins to cause problems in the person with a suppressed immune system, and then it can infect wounds or enter the lungs and resist treatment. MRSA can be passed on by skin contact but will only colonise other people if they have a compromised immune system.

Relevance to massage

Healthy massage therapists don't know if they carry the MRSA bacteria, but maybe should act as if they do when taking hygiene precautions, particularly when treating a client with an auto-immune disorder or someone taking medication that suppresses the immune system. This includes washing hands thoroughly before and after treatment, and also paying attention to door handles and toilet handles. These are places where the bacteria could linger, and which are used by a number of clients throughout the day. It is recommended to clean them regularly with disinfectant wipes.

Trauma

Trauma is the word for any mechanical or chemical injury to the body. A fractured radius after a fall, a whiplash injury from a car crash, or repetitive strain injury from occupational use are all examples of mechanical trauma. Exposure to chemicals, pollution and poisons, on the skin or taken internally, are examples of chemical trauma. Prolonged or severe emotional disturbance may also have a traumatic effect on body tissues. Most musculoskeletal problems we treat are traumatic in origin, either through injury or repetitive use.

Degenerative conditions

All the body tissues gradually change as we age. These changes are not, in themselves, disorders but are part of the normal process of ageing. Skin loses its suppleness, becoming thinner, and, in extreme old age, it is likely to tear easily. Fascia becomes less pliable, tendons and ligaments tighten, and the range of motion in joints decreases. Rate of nerve transmission slows down, and with it our reactions to events. Sight and hearing become less acute.

All of these things can be adjusted to, but there are some degenerative processes that cause discomfort and suffering. The most common ones are osteoarthritis, affecting joints, and osteoporosis, which affects bone. After the age of 50, most of us will notice changes in our body brought about by the normal ageing process.

Other causes of disease

Apart from these major categories, there are also those conditions that are genetically determined, which include haemophilia, cystic fibrosis and sickle cell anaemia, and those that are caused by, or are side effects of, medical intervention, such as the adhesions that can occur in the fascia after major surgery, causing pain and discomfort.

Failure of the immune system accounts for another large group of problems, ranging from the common and annoying (but not usually life-threatening) allergies, to much more serious conditions, such as cancers, rheumatoid arthritis and lupus. Much research is still needed to properly understand these auto-immune failures.

Chapter 6
Musculoskeletal disorders

TRAUMATIC CONDITIONS OF THE MUSCULOSKELETAL SYSTEM

This section looks at the common musculoskeletal problems resulting from trauma that we come across as massage therapists, and considerations for working with them. Specialist remedial or sports massage techniques aren't described, but common sense ways that the non-specialist massage therapist can adapt her work to each condition.

Fractures

Breaks in bones vary from hairline cracks to complete breaks with bony parts penetrating through the skin. They can happen throughout life, but are more common in young people, due to injuries sustained in the physical activities of this age group, or in the elderly whose bones are thinner and weaker. In between those ages, most fractures result from sports activity or vehicle accidents.

Fractures are painful and involve some reduction of

movement at the nearest joint. There are three main types: partial fractures in which the bone is not completely broken, simple fractures where there is a clean break that does not damage surrounding tissues or the skin, and compound fractures, where the broken ends protrude through soft tissues and the skin.

There are many further classifications. In comminuted fractures, the bone splinters at the break; in impacted fractures, the broken bones ends have been pushed into one another. A greenstick fracture occurs in children whose bones are not completely ossified. There is bending and partial fracture of the bone, similar to the breaking of a green twig.

Recommendations for massage

A fracture is a local contraindication to massage while healing, and may anyway be inaccessible inside plaster or a splint.

Broken bone can take months to heal, depending on the type of fracture, the size of the bone, and the age and general health of the person. Older people's bones heal less quickly. The rest of the body can be massaged normally, assuming there are no other complications. Pay attention to parts of the body that have been overused to compensate for the restriction caused by the fracture. Avoid getting oil near plaster casts, because this can soften them.

Once the bone is well set, gentle massage of muscles adjacent to the fracture may be attempted, but remember that the surrounding muscles will be atrophied and weak through lack of use. Do not exert pressure on the site of the fracture.

Sprains and strains

A sprain refers to damage to ligaments when they are forced past their normal range of movement. The most common sprain is a twisted ankle, followed by injuries to the ligaments of the sacroiliac joint and the fingers and knees, these last ones being common with sports people. The damage can be chronic or acute, and can range from a few torn fibres, to a complete tear.

The tissue around sprained ligaments swells up and is painful. Stretching may cause them to become flabby, and the joint they support to become unstable. Muscles surrounding a sprain will tend to tighten to protect the joint, and, even after the ligaments have healed, the muscles may stay tight and overworking.

Strain is damage to muscle tissue or tendon that occurs when a muscle is subjected to excessive or violent sudden force, either when it is contracting or when it is being stretched. Strains are usually less serious than sprains. Firstly, muscles have good blood supply and therefore heal much more quickly, and secondly, there is less chance of damage to a joint as well.

Strains range from a mild condition, where a few muscle fibres are torn and there is a little bleeding, to the situation in which much of the muscle tissue and the surrounding sheath are torn, and there is considerable bleeding. In the most serious strains, there is complete rupture of the muscle. This is very serious, causes extreme pain and requires hospital treatment.

Recommendations for massage

Do not attempt to massage acute sprains or strains. Unless you have specific training in sports injury massage, you should not massage the area affected in any of these conditions immediately after injury.

Never massage over areas of bruising, which, as an indicator of internal muscle injury with internal bleeding or fluid seepage, would be aggravated by massage. Mild injuries may be treated after 48 hours, using massage to improve circulation to the area and reduce general muscle stiffness. Passive movements of joints adjacent to the injury are helpful to maintain mobility.

Draining strokes can be helpful to disperse swelling, but if in doubt about the appropriateness of massage, consult with a sports trainer or physiotherapist. When a joint is sprained, the surrounding muscles attempt to take over the job of the damaged ligaments, and may become very tense. Even after the ligaments have healed, the muscles may have become habituated to this role. Massage of these muscles is beneficial.

Both sprains and strains that result in the tearing of tissue can give rise to scarring as part of the healing process. Since scar tissue lacks flexibility, the functioning of affected ligaments or muscles is impaired. In the case of ligaments, scarring can lead to further injuries unless it is treated by a professional trained to deal with sports injuries – a sports masseur, trainer, or physiotherapist. After a strain, the scarred muscle may also remain tight to protect the damaged area even when this is no longer needed. Massage of chronic scars using transverse friction strokes, and of the residual holding patterns in muscles using kneading, draining and percussion, is very beneficial.

Herniated or 'slipped' disc

As one ages, the fibres of the inter-vertebral discs can become worn and tear under pressure, especially if there is excessive or sudden strain on the spine. A 'slipped disc' then occurs when part of the central pulp becomes displaced, bulging out to one side, and putting pressure on the spinal cord and the nerve roots as they emerge from the spine. This can appear to happen very suddenly without any obvious cause, although the affected disc may have been degenerating for some time. Since the cartilage of the disc has no nerve supply, there are no warning signals. The lumbar spine is most likely to be affected, with severe back pain and tenderness, and pain may be referred down the legs as well. Doctors usually recommend bed rest and painkillers. In extreme cases surgery is considered, either to remove the pulp of the disc or to fuse the vertebrae together.

People sometimes refer to any sharp back pain as a slipped disc, but an actual slipped disc is very painful and debilitating. If the pain in the spinal muscles near the site is on one side only, this is more likely to be a trapped nerve, which massage may ease. If the pain is on both sides of the spine, it is more likely to be a slipped disc, in which case refer the client to an osteopath, chiropractor or physiotherapist.

Recommendations for massage

In the acute stage refer to an osteopath or chiropractor for treatment. When the most acute stage has subsided, gentle massage, sensitively applied, may help to relieve pain from associated muscle spasms. Relaxation massage to the head, hands and feet may bring some relief from pain.

OVERUSE CONDITIONS OF THE MUSCULOSKELETAL SYSTEM

Repetitive strain injury (RSI)

This refers to any chronic, painful and debilitating overuse condition. It is a term that has only recently been given recognised status, as a result of legal cases claiming compensation for injuries received in an occupational setting.

Carpal tunnel syndrome

This is the most common type of repetitive strain injury. It can occur as a result of occupational injury, such as prolonged typing, but it can also be one of the complications of pregnancy. The tendons from the muscles of the forearm that flex the fingers pass under a band of fibrous tissue on the front of the wrist – the carpal tunnel.

Overuse or regular awkward use of these muscles can inflame the tissue and cause the tendons to swell, putting pressure on the nerves and blood vessels that also pass through here. The result can be weakness and numbness or tingling in the hands.

Frozen shoulder

The socket of the shoulder joint is shallow, to allow for a large range of movement. The muscles and the ligaments that surround the joint provide stability. Damage to them causes pain and instinctive restriction when movement is attempted, and is called a frozen shoulder. Inflammation may occur in any muscle or tendon separately, in which case only the movement initiated by that muscle would be affected.

Bursitis

When a bursa, a small fluid-filled sac in a joint to reduce friction, becomes inflamed through pressure, friction or injury, the condition known as bursitis develops. There is pain that is aggravated by movement. Deltoid bursitis is common in tennis players and gymnasts. Housemaid's knee refers to inflammation of any of the bursae in the knee joint. The other more common problem sites are the shoulder joint (sub-acromial bursitis) and the base of the big toe (bunions).

Tendinitis

The strain of a tendon, often at the junction with the muscle or with the periosteum, gives rise to inflammation, pain and stiffness. As the tendon recovers, scar tissue will be formed, which is less stretchable than the original material and susceptible to re-injury. Tennis elbow is tendinitis of the muscles of the back of the forearm at their insertion, and is caused by excessive hammering or sawing-type movements, or a tense, awkward grip on a tennis racquet. The Achilles tendon is also susceptible to strains. At the insertion with the calcaneus is a bursa that can become inflamed. Both of these problems can occur in runners who wear inadequate footwear.

Recommendations for massage

In the acute phase very gentle mobilisation of the affected and adjacent joints is indicated to prevent loss of movement. When the inflammation has subsided, massage of surrounding muscles may help to relieve pain, and prevent immobilisation if a joint is involved. It helps to massage parts of the body that may be compensating. In the case of tendinitis, cross friction strokes, moving the fingers across the direction of the tendon fibres, can help with the healing.

DEGENERATIVE CONDITIONS OF THE MUSCULOSKELETAL SYSTEM

Arthritis and rheumatism

These terms are often used interchangeably in everyday language to refer to pain connected with movement. Arthritis means inflammation of joints – with pain, stiffness and loss of movement – whilst rheumatism usually refers to aches or pains that come from muscles, tendons or ligaments, as well as from joints. Arthritis can be a secondary condition arising from other diseases; there is a form associated with psoriasis, for example. There are many varieties of arthritis: three of the most common forms are described here.

Osteoarthritis

This is a very common condition, affecting almost everyone over the age of 60 to some extent, but to varying degrees. For the majority of people, this may be experienced merely as stiff joints. For some, the symptoms include pain, stiffness and swelling, leading to reduced movement as the condition worsens. It usually develops slowly, and, in the more advanced stages, joints may become inflamed.

Osteoarthritis is caused by wear and tear of the hyaline cartilage. It is made worse by previous injury or excessive pressure on the joint in overweight people. As the cartilage thins with age, cracks appear and penetrate to the bone underneath. Bony growths can also develop. Weight-bearing joints, such as the hip and the knee, are most often affected, as well as fingers (which may not be painful) and the spine.

Recommendations for massage

Massage is locally contraindicated if joints are inflamed. Otherwise, relaxation massage can be beneficial in providing some pain relief, and gentle mobilisation and stretching of the joints may prevent further deterioration, provided more care is taken with painful joints. Kneading and draining muscles surrounding affected joints reduces stiffness and aids circulation.

Rheumatoid arthritis

This form of arthritis is not a degenerative condition, but is included here, because of the potential confusion with osteoarthritis. Clients will be very clear about which sort they have – you won't have to make a diagnosis. This one is an auto-immune disease, in which the immune system attacks the body's own tissues. This chronic disease can cause inflammation of many parts of the body. The skin, lungs, eyes and internal organs may all be affected as well as the joints, and sometimes also muscles, tendons and blood vessels. It is not necessarily constant but can regularly flare up and then die down.

The joints most affected are usually the hands and feet, often on both sides of the body at once, and sometimes the neck. Inside the joint, the synovial membrane becomes inflamed, the fluid builds up and the joint swells. If it progresses, which only happens in a proportion of people, the cartilage and then the bone is affected until, over time, the joint may become deformed and the parts may fuse together.

Recommendations for massage

Since stress may be a predisposing factor to the disease flaring up, massage for relaxation is beneficial and can reduce discomfort.

In the early stages, careful joint mobilisation and massage around joints to reduce stiffening in the soft tissues are helpful to maintain mobility in the joints. In the later stages, stretches or manipulations of the spine are contra-indicated, particularly in the cervical region, because this could disturb or break bony fusions that may have developed between the vertebrae.

Be aware that clients who are on painkillers may have reduced sensation and be less able to give accurate feedback about pressure or range of movement.

Ankylosing spondylitis

This type of arthritis, involving inflammation and ossification of the inter-vertebral discs of the spine and the sacroiliac joints, leads to stiff and sometimes fused joints, often slightly flexed. It is an inherited auto-immune disease that mostly affects men in their mid-teens to mid-thirties.

Most commonly, it starts as lower back pain, made worse by rest, and stiffness, especially around the sacrum. It may stay here, although sometimes it progresses up the spine, and occasionally affects joints outside the spine. It can flare up at times, and there may also be inflammation of the lungs, heart, eyes and other organs. Osteoporosis may be present as well.

Recommendations for massage

In acute phases, massage is contraindicated in areas of pain and inflammation. At other times, work under a doctor's supervision. Take care to negotiate the use of supports to give maximum comfort.

Gentle massage of the back and limbs may give pain relief, and, in the early stages, help maintain some mobility. Do not put pressure on muscles near the spine, as they may be involved in protective splinting of the vulnerable areas, and because osteoporosis may be present.

Osteoporosis

Osteoporosis, or 'brittle bones,' is fairly common among elderly people, particularly women after the menopause. Predisposing factors include low body-weight, a history of anorexia in adolescence, smoking and lack of weight-bearing exercise.

Bone density reduces gradually and this condition is often only diagnosed when the first fracture occurs. The calcium content of the bone reduces, and the bones become soft and crumbly, and liable to break easily on sudden impact, especially in the wrist and hip. There may be chronic back pain and, in the advanced stages, the vertebrae may collapse.

Recommendations for massage

Known osteoporotic areas are local contraindications. Negotiate comfortable positions and the use of supports with the person. Take particular care in getting the client on and off the table, because this is probably where any damage could occur, were the client to fall.

Massage on the rest of the body should be gentle, with no stretches, joint manipulations or use of percussive strokes, or use of heavy pressure over bones. The main intention is to help the client relax.

Always be cautious with pressure when massaging an older person, particularly women, as they may unknowingly have osteoporosis.

Osteomalacia and rickets

Vitamin D deficiency results in the softening and swelling of the bones. In adults this is called osteomalacia; in children, rickets. If undetected, this condition results in bow legs and a 'necklace' of thickenings at the sternocostal junctions. Vitamin D is present in a balanced diet, and also produced in the body through exposure to sunlight.

Recommendations for massage

These are the same as those described for osteoporosis.

OTHER CONDITIONS AFFECTING BONES, MUSCLES AND JOINTS

Spinal curvature

The spine has natural curves for resilience – a convex curve between the shoulders and concave curves in the neck and lower back. We all have small postural imbalances, but they become problematic when these curves become exaggerated and rigidify into unbalanced positions. This can occur for a number of reasons. Inherited factors, accidents, disease or poor posture over a long time are a few. The underlying physical cause may be muscular, in which case massage may help to remedy the curvature, or due to connective tissue or bony changes, in which case the aim of massage would be to reduce general discomfort and tension in the muscles.

Kyphosis

Kyphosis is a pronounced curve in the upper spine, commonly called a hunchback. The rhomboids, long spinal muscles, and trapezius are stretched and weak, while the neck extensors, intercostals and pectorals are shortened and strong. The head and scapulae are pulled forward.

Scoliosis

This is a pronounced curve in the spine to one side. One shoulder or hip will be higher than the other. This condition is more common in adolescence and in girls. If the cause is structural, the underlying problem is muscular, but if it is functional scoliosis, the cause is skeletal. In cases of severe skeletal scoliosis, surgery is done to correct the curvature, sometimes implanting a rod beside the spine. Spinal muscles on one side are stretched and weak, and, on the other, contracted and tight.

Lordosis

This is an excessive curve in the lower back, or swayback. Abdominal muscles are weak and the back muscles are tight to compensate.

Recommendations for massage

When working with clients who have pronounced spinal curvatures, be prepared for the possibility that their movement may be limited. They may not be able to lie flat on their back or stomach, and you will need to adapt your techniques and body use accordingly. Use cushions or pillows to ensure they have adequate support. Massage of the back should avoid pressure on the spine, and aim to tonify weak muscles and relax tight ones. Leg and hip muscle groups may be tense as they compensate for postural problems, and appreciate general massage.

Cramp

Cramp is an involuntary contraction of a muscle, usually accompanied by pain, which occurs mostly in the calf muscles and sometimes in the forearm muscles. It is commonly caused by lack of oxygen to a muscle, either through overworking the muscle or because of chronic tension in the muscle that is impeding the blood supply. It can also be due to, or aggravated by, a lack of calcium or magnesium or, in hot climates, of salt.

Recommendations for massage

In the immediate situation, stretch the muscle to relieve the cramp. Be wary of doing massage on the muscle until it has calmed down. When the cramp has reduced, massage can help the muscle to relax, and, in the long-term, regular massage and stretching exercises should reduce the likelihood of further episodes.

Muscle spasm

Muscles can have longer-term involuntary muscle spasms that ache rather than give a sharp pain. These too can be symptoms of muscle overuse, in which case treat them in the same way as for cramp. However, such spasms also commonly occur when muscles tighten to protect injuries or to reduce movement in painful joints. If the client's history indicates that this could be the case, don't apply pressure, and be careful when doing passive movements.

Fibrosis

This term refers to the scarring that forms in any tissue when the damage is so extensive that there is too little healthy tissue to make good the repair. Scar tissue is stronger than the original and has little flexibility. In muscles the causes range from severe strains to chronic muscular tension.

Recommendations for massage

Kneading and draining strokes in the muscle tissue around the scar and of the adjacent muscles and antagonists, to improve circulation and reduce tension, are indicated. Cross fibre fiction on the scar tissue itself is also helpful.

Fibrositis, fibromyositis and fibromyalgia

These are all terms for a condition of unknown origin, with varying symptoms that include fatigue, sleep disorders, digestive problems and muscle weakness and pain. Joints may also be stiff and swollen. It is most common in women between 25 and 45 years.

Recommendations for massage

Take a case history each time, since your client's symptoms will vary from session to session, and alter your treatment accordingly. Gentle whole-body massage, using rhythmic strokes, is indicated. Avoid working deeply, or for too long, both of which could tire an already fatigued system.

Muscular dystrophy

There are four kinds of muscular dystrophy, which is a neuromuscular disease. They are inherited and cause symmetrical and progressive weakening and degeneration of muscle, for which there is no cure. They differ in their onset and severity, and two kinds affect only men. There is no loss of sensation.

Recommendations for massage

Clients with muscle-wasting conditions take longer to do ordinary things, such as getting undressed or climbing on a table. Make allowances for this. Massage that helps circulation, and passive joint movements, may slow down muscle atrophy. Since these conditions also affect smooth muscle, there may be problems with peristalsis. If your client is constipated, abdominal massage may help.

Myasthenia gravis

This disease of the immune system affects nerve impulses to

the muscles, resulting in muscle weakness and fatigue. The limb muscles and those to do with speech, swallowing and chewing are most affected. There is no loss of sensation.

Recommendations for massage

The same considerations apply as described above, for the muscular dystrophies. Gentle massage may help to relieve pain or muscle spasm. Clients with myasthenia gravis may be taking steroids, which reduce immune-system functioning, so take care not to expose the client to infection.

Chapter 7
Skin disorders

Dermatology is the name given to the study, diagnosis and treatment of skin disorders, some of which, like eczema, are very common and some very rare. There are so many types of rashes, spots, lesions and sores that it can be quite hard for a doctor in general practice to identify a skin condition accurately, so we certainly shouldn't have expectations that we can tell our massage clients about their skin problems. However, it is important to know the names of the common disorders and whether or not a condition is contagious. Usually, someone with a chronic skin condition, one which is ongoing or recurring, will know its name, and will be able to give you information about it. Undiagnosed conditions require that you follow common-sense guidelines for massage and refer your client to a doctor.

General guidelines

When a medical condition is described as contagious, it means that it is an infection that is transmitted through direct skin contact, compared to an infection that is transmitted in food, water or breathed in from the air. Impetigo is a contagious condition, for example, but salmonella and viral pneumonia are not. However, not all skin infections are contagious. You can't 'catch' spots or infected cuts although they do contain bacteria and are local contraindications. Areas of skin that are bleeding, broken or weeping fluid are also local contraindications, because body fluids (blood, lymph, pus) may contain infectious agents, which could be transmitted to the therapist or other parts of the client's body, if there are cuts or openings in the skin. Cuts on the therapist's hands and arms should be covered by a plaster or finger cot for this reason. Finger cots look like mini condoms and are useful if a whole finger or thumb needs to be covered. They are available from good chemists.

The general recommendation for most contagious skin conditions is that if only a small area is affected, it should be treated as a local contraindication, but if the area is extensive then it is advisable not to massage at all until the condition has been successfully treated.

Hygiene is particularly important when treating clients with contagious skin conditions. If you use paper roll covering over a couch cover, it might be advisable to change the fabric couch cover as well as the paper cover. Always use clean towels and disinfect couch surfaces regularly.

The psychological aspect of treating a client with a skin condition, particularly a severe or chronic one, needs to be taken into account. A person with chronic eczema, say, may feel very sensitive or embarrassed about the appearance of her skin, especially if she has had eczema since childhood and may have endured bullying or teasing, or been excluded from activities as a result. Such a person may be concerned that you might find her skin ugly, or be repulsed, or that you may not want to touch it, and may need reassurance. Many conditions are not contraindications to massage, but ask permission and negotiate with your client. Don't assume that it's just fine to massage.

BACTERIAL INFECTIONS

Acne vulgaris

This is commonly found in teenagers whose hormonal changes increase sebaceous gland activity, and sebum builds up in the pores. Bacterial infection then causes whiteheads, which are accumulations of sebum, pus and dead cells, and inflammation. Severe acne can leave scarring.

Recommendations for massage

Acne is not contagious, so can be massaged over if not severe, inflamed or weeping. Be careful to avoid creams or lotions that might clog the pores further.

Boils and carbuncles

These are caused by staphylococcal infection round a hair root or sweat gland, with pain, swelling and formation of pus. A carbuncle is a collection of boils.

Recommendations for massage

Boils and carbuncles are local contraindications although massaging the surrounding areas may help healing by improving circulation flow.

Impetigo

Most commonly found in children, impetigo is typified by raised fluid-filled sores and crusts on the face, particularly round the mouth and nose.

Recommendations for massage

The fluid contained in the sores is highly infectious, so this condition is a total contraindication if the sores are weeping, and if the person has not started medical treatment.

If the sores have dried, treat impetigo as a local contraindication, avoid the area and take particular care with hygiene precautions.

VIRAL INFECTIONS

Herpes simplex

The herpes simplex virus causes clusters of sore blisters. There are two kinds – cold sores round the mouth, and genital herpes that are transmitted sexually. Once present in the body this virus cannot be removed. It lies dormant, and erupts in times of stress. When active, the virus is contagious.

Recommendations for massage

Cold sores on the face are a local contraindication. There is no reason not to massage someone with genital herpes, but if the virus is active, the client may prefer to keep his or her underwear on. The virus can survive outside the body for a few hours, so extra care is needed with hygiene.

Warts and verrucas

The human papilloma virus causes the small, rough, non-malignant tumours called warts. More than half of all warts clear up after a few years without treatment. Verrucas are warts on the soles of the feet.

Recommendations for massage

Small warts and verruccas are local contraindications to massage, but if large areas are affected, it is advisable to avoid massage.

FUNGAL INFECTIONS

Ringworm

A worm does not, as the name implies, cause ringworm, although it does look as if a little worm has burrowed a red, itchy shiny circle under the skin.

Recommendations for massage

If large areas of the body are affected, this is a total contraindication because the condition is contagious. If only a small area is affected and can be covered, it is a local contraindication. Take particular care with hygiene precautions.

Athlete's foot

This is a common, itchy infection between the toes.

Recommendations for massage

Athlete's foot is a local contraindication.

Candida

Candida, or thrush, is a yeast-like fungus that grows on the mucous membranes of the intestines, vagina, and mouth, as well as on the skin. It becomes red and scaly, and there may be white discharge.

Recommendations for massage

As for ringworm, if larger areas on the skin are affected, treat as a total contraindication, otherwise avoid the infected patches and take extra hygiene precautions.

PARASITES

Scabies

The tiny mite responsible for scabies crawls under the skin to lay its eggs. It is commonly found on the wrists, between the fingers, or on the genitals.

Recommendations for massage

Scabies is so highly contagious that it can be caught from infected linen after the client has left. It is definitely a total contraindication until it has cleared up. However, it is so extremely itchy that it is unlikely a scabies sufferer could lie still enough for a massage!

Head lice, nits and fleas

The blood-sucking lice, with a preference for the head (there are other varieties that prefer the pubic area), and their white eggs ('nits') are easily transmitted, as are fleas. Fleas tend not to live on the human body, but head lice are increasingly common in young school children and people associated with them. Nits look like tiny grains of sugar attached to the base of the hair.

Recommendations for massage

Lice and nits are total contraindications until cleared up, to protect the practitioner. If the client is unaware that she is infected and you notice lice or nits during the treatment, use your discretion. Either stop the massage and explain why, or continue, avoiding the head area, and put all linen in the wash immediately afterwards.

NON-INFECTIOUS CONDITIONS

Dermatitis and eczema

These terms refer to a group of diseases characterised by

inflammation of the skin with redness, itching or burning, and, at times, weeping, blistering or formation of scales. Some authorities group them all together, while others see eczema as a constitutional condition, one that arises from within, and dermatitis as an occupational one. Thus, contact dermatitis is skin inflammation caused by contact with a chemical, such as washing powder, perfume, metals or fabric dye, or certain plants. Atopic eczema, which often starts in childhood, is likely to occur alongside allergies such as hay fever and asthma. Other types of eczema include varicose eczema, which is scaling and brown discoloration in the ankles and lower legs, usually due to poor circulation but not necessarily associated with varicose veins. Dandruff is a form of eczema, occurring only on the scalp.

Psoriasis

The cause of psoriasis is unknown. It is a chronic condition where the epidermal cells grow too fast and reach the surface of the skin without being properly keratinised. The cells clump together to form thick red scaly plaques. There are many types, each affecting different body areas. The most common sort affects the elbows, knees, scalp and back. Sunlight seems to help.

Recommendations for massage

Assuming the skin is not broken or weeping, neither eczema, dermatitis nor psoriasis are contraindications. Be aware that scales may dislodge. Massage may even be beneficial, but ask the client if he would like you to work on, or avoid, affected areas. Ask also about medical treatment. If the client is using steroid creams, there may be thinning of the skin. (See below for general recommendations for 'thin skin'.)

Cellulitis

This bacterial infection involves swelling, pain and redness of large areas of skin, often in the legs. The sufferer often has a temperature and flu-like symptoms and would be too unwell to come for a treatment.

OTHER MILD/COMMON NON-INFECTIOUS SKIN CONDITIONS

Bruising

Internal superficial bleeding causes the sometimes spectacular changes in colour of a bruise. Bruises can be painful.

Recommendations for massage

Recent or severe bruises are local contraindications. Check with your client. Massage of the surrounding areas may help healing by bringing nutrients to, and removing wastes from, the area.

Blisters

Blisters are caused by an accumulation of lymph below the surface of the skin, in response to friction or pressure on a specific spot.

Recommendations for massage

Blisters are local contraindications.

Bedsores/pressure sores

Commonly affecting people who are bedridden, or who wear casts or braces, pressure sores occur when an area of skin is subjected to continuous pressure, the blood supply to the area is cut off and cells begin to die.

Recommendations for massage

Pressure sores are a local contraindication, but gentle massage of surrounding areas may help improve circulation.

Vitiligo

Vitiligo is a disorder of the melanin pigment in the skin, and may be an auto-immune problem. Patches of skin lose their colour and their protection against the sun's rays. This condition appears more obvious in darker-skinned people.

Recommendations for massage

Vitiligo is not a contraindication.

Liver or age spots

The brown spots found on the skin of older people, particularly the back of the hand, are not contraindications to massage.

Skin tags

Skin tags are small harmless growths attached to the skin by a tiny stalk, or peduncle, and are common in older people.

Recommendations for massage

Skin tags are not a contraindication, but avoid vigorous massage or friction that could break the stalks and cause bleeding.

Stretch marks

Stretch marks are the white lines caused by sudden stretching of the skin as a result of pregnancy, weight gain, or bodybuilding.

Recommendations for massage

Deep massage or friction is contraindicated over stretch marks. (See 'thin skin'.)

Skin cancer

Skin cancer is the most common form of cancer, and the quickest to diagnose, since it is visible on the surface of the body. The massage therapist is in a good position to notice moles, lumps or patches of skin, which darken in colour, grow rapidly, or bleed or ulcerate, and can bring these to the attention of the client. While there are many harmless reasons for changes in lumps on the skin, there is always a small possibility that a growth may be cancerous, particularly in a person with a history of overexposure to the sun.

There are three main kinds – basal cell carcinoma (rodent ulcer), which grows quite slowly, and squamous cell carcinoma and malignant melanoma, both of which develop rapidly. Kaposi's sarcoma is a rare form of skin cancer found in people with AIDS.

Recommendations for massage

Massage is generally beneficial for people with cancer. Although it is true that some cancers are spread through the lymphatic system, and that massage may affect the flow of lymph, there is no evidence that massage can spread cancer cells. Massage can provide a valuable source of comfort and relief from emotional stress. Having said that, all skin cancers are local contraindications until removed and treatment is finished. Radiation, one form of treatment, causes thinning of the skin. (See below and 'massage for people with cancer'.)

Thin skin

If the blood supply to the skin becomes restricted, for whatever reason, nourishment fails to reach the epidermal cells and the rate of growth slows down. The cells that produce collagen and elastin, the fibres that give the skin its elasticity, die through lack of food and oxygen. The skin becomes thin and papery, less elastic and liable to tear easily. This is a normal occurrence as we become very old, but is also the result of prolonged use of steroid creams or radiation treatment. Varicose veins or areas of chronic oedema may be covered by thin skin, as are large areas of scar tissue from burns, injury or surgical treatment.

Recommendations for massage

Massage over areas of thin skin should be gentle. With a very elderly person, the whole body should be treated with gentle massage, but, in other thin skin conditions, gentle massage may only be required locally. For example, a young, fit athlete with a patch of thin skin on the site of an old burn can be massaged without precautions except over the thin skin area. What does gentle massage mean? It is obvious that the holding and light contact strokes (light vibration, stroking, light effleurage) could be considered gentle massage, but all the other techniques could also be performed in a gentle way, with the exception of percussion, friction or twisting techniques, which could tear the skin.

Chapter 8
Cardiovascular disorders

When a new client arrives and says that he suffers from a heart condition, or that he has a blood disorder, our anxiety levels may rise. Is it safe to massage? Should we ask the client to go away and get a doctor's letter? Should we use gentle massage only?

The disorders of the circulatory system range from those that are exacerbated by stress and therefore benefit from relaxing massage, to those that are potentially fatal and may be total contraindications. Angina is an example of the first, and deep vein thrombosis (DVT) comes in the second category. But the situation isn't that simple – there is also a form of angina that is a contraindication for massage because the sufferer is at risk of heart attack. In the case of DVT, massage would be a local contraindication if the DVT was controlled by medication. An additional problem for the non-medical practitioner is the terminology. What's the difference between arteriosclerosis and artherosclerosis? When is a clot called an embolism and when is it a thrombosis?

Probably more so than any other system, disorders of the

circulatory system are a minefield when it comes to massage! As a general rule, when treating someone with a cardiovascular disorder, you should notify the client's doctor and ask him/her to contact you if there are any concerns.

To clarify the complexity, it is helpful to think of circulatory disorders as those that affect the blood itself, those that affect the circulation of the blood and lymph, those that affect the arteries, veins and capillaries, and those that are to do with the heart. Furthermore, within the last two categories, some disorders are due to problems with the structure of the blood vessels or heart, and others are caused by obstructions within the blood vessels or heart, which interfere with free circulation of the blood.

In healthy people, there are two considerations for massage relating to the circulatory system. One is that you never put heavy or prolonged pressure on the major superficial arteries. These are the arteries on the inner surface of the elbow joint and on the back of the knee, and the two arteries where you feel for a pulse (the carotid artery at the side of the neck and the ulnar artery on the inner surface of the wrist). The other is that, when massaging the limbs with firm pressure, always work towards the heart. Massaging in the opposite direction poses the risk of turning the valves in the veins inside out and permanently damaging them.

DISORDERS OF THE BLOOD

Anaemia

Anaemia refers to a number of conditions in which the

capacity of the blood to carry oxygen to the tissues is reduced. There may be insufficient red blood cells or insufficient haemoglobin. It is a sign of an underlying disorder. Pernicious anaemia arises from lack of vitamin B12, and iron-deficient anaemia, as the title suggests, from lack of iron. A person who is anaemic may look pale, feel tired, be susceptible to the cold, and lack concentration. Sickle cell anaemia is an inherited form of anaemia found in peoples of Black African descent. The red blood cells, instead of being circular, are sickle-shaped, which reduces the surface for carrying oxygen. Thalassaemia is another inherited form of anaemia common to people of Turkish or Cypriot descent. Both these conditions can result in joint pain as well as the symptoms listed previously.

Recommendations for massage

Relaxing massage is beneficial, since it will help the client rest, but the level of vitality of the person at the time of massage would determine the quality of treatment. If the client is very fatigued, give gentle massage only. If the anaemia is caused by an underlying bleeding disorder, do not use any excessive pressure at all.

Leukaemia

Leukaemia, or blood cancer, develops when immature white blood cells in the bone marrow and lymphatic tissue multiply excessively, interfering with the ability of normal white cells and platelets to do their work. General immunity to disease and blood-clotting ability are compromised. There are different types, but all sufferers are more prone to infection and bleed easily. The liver and spleen may be enlarged.

Recommendations for massage

Consult with the medical practitioner first about the advisability of massage. Use gentle massage, avoiding the abdomen. Do not treat if you have an infection, such as a cold, yourself. (See also 'massage for people with cancer'.)

Haemophilia

This inherited disorder is a failure of the blood to clot properly because one or more of the factors needed for the clotting process to work properly is missing. There is a mild form, where problematic bleeding only happens after a severe trauma, a moderate form, and a severe form where the individual may bleed spontaneously under the skin or into joints.

Recommendations for massage

Severe haemophilia is a total contraindication to massage. With mild forms, consult with the medical practitioner first about the advisability of massage. Use very gentle massage and help the client on and off the table.

DISORDERS OF THE CIRCULATION

Hypertension

Blood pressure depends on the ability of the heart to pump

blood round the body, the volume of blood to be pumped, and the size of the arteries, whose muscular walls can dilate or constrict. These factors interact to adjust blood pressure to the different needs of the body over time, but sometimes this mechanism goes wrong.

Hypertension, or high blood pressure, is common and often there are no symptoms. It can result from kidney disorders or arteriosclerosis, but, in the majority of cases, there is no known cause. It has been linked to stress, smoking, obesity, lack of exercise and genetic factors. If not controlled by medication, hypertension can lead to damage of the heart or brain in the long term.

Recommendations for massage

Deep abdominal massage is contraindicated, but relaxing massage is probably beneficial for someone with high blood pressure, to keep stress levels down. If someone has high blood pressure that is not controlled by medication, diet or exercise, consult with the medical practitioner first about the advisability of massage. If the client is taking medication, he may experience hypotension after a relaxing massage.

Hypotension

Hypotension, or low blood pressure, is not considered a medical problem and there are no massage considerations. However, after the treatment, ask the client to sit up slowly and take care helping them off the table, because the change in position from lying to sitting may cause the person to faint.

Oedema

Oedema is an accumulation of fluid in the tissues, caused by failure of the lymphatic system to drain properly. The area is swollen, and there may be pain and heaviness. If you press a finger into the tissue, an indentation remains for a short time.

Oedema may be a sign of a serious underlying condition, such as heart failure, kidney failure or liver disease, or it may develop if lymph glands are removed as part of treatment for cancer. It may be temporary and have much milder causes, for example localised inflammation. The swollen ankles commonly experienced by pregnant women are also caused by oedema.

Recommendations for massage

Massage of someone with generalised oedema resulting from a serious condition should only be carried out after consultation with their doctor. For most of the common types of oedema light massage is probably beneficial, if it can help stimulate a sluggish lymphatic circulation. Supports under affected limbs to assist drainage are recommended. Use draining strokes on areas closer to the torso than the oedema to free up the lymph ducts before working on the affected areas. For example, if the ankles are swollen, work on the thighs and calves first. Anyone with chronic oedema is likely to have thin skin in the affected areas: use gentle massage and be sensitive to the person's feelings about their condition. Manual lymphatic drainage (MLD) is a specialised type of massage, which works specifically with the lymphatic system and is particularly helpful in treating oedema.

Raynaud's disease

As part of the fight or flight response, the small arteries supplying blood to the periphery of the body constrict to divert blood to the muscles. This also happens when it is very cold, to conserve heat. In a person with Raynaud's disease this reaction is abnormal, particularly in the hands and feet, which can suddenly go cold and tingling. The condition may last for a few minutes at a time, or may be chronic.

Recommendations for massage

Massage of the limbs is beneficial because it can help restore blood flow to the hands and feet. Relaxing massage helps because it lowers sympathetic nervous system activity.

DISORDERS OF THE BLOOD VESSELS

Varicose veins

Varicose veins develop when the valves, which prevent the backflow of blood against gravity, are damaged and pockets of blood accumulate in the vein, causing the thin walls to stretch and bulge. This is a common problem in the superficial veins in the legs. The symptoms are bulging knobbly veins just under the surface of the skin, and heavy, aching legs.

Support stockings relieve discomfort but treatment is to strip the affected veins out, or to block them. The process of returning blood to the heart is then taken over by the deep veins. If untreated, fluid accumulates around the ankles, and they swell. The skin can become discoloured and the veins ulcerated. Pregnancy, obesity and inheritance are risk factors, but the real cause is prolonged standing.

Recommendations for massage

Locate the varicose veins before your client lies down, because they can be harder to identify in the supine position. Massage is contraindicated in the area directly over, or immediately below, varicose veins. The affected area can be held gently while the rest of the leg is massaged. Use draining strokes on the thigh above the affected area first, to decongest the area and assist blood flow. Support under the legs to aid drainage back to the heart during massage is recommended.

Blood clots

Thrombosis is the term for a clot that is attached to the wall of a vein or, more rarely, an artery. Small clots in superficial veins don't usually cause any problems. Large clots in the deep veins of the legs are the ones that can detach and travel in the circulation to the lungs, heart or brain, with potentially fatal consequences. A travelling clot is called an embolism, but embolism also refers to any foreign material, such as air or fatty tissue from a bone fracture, in the circulation. Clots are treated with anti-coagulants, which help them to disperse.

Thrombophlebitis

If a superficial vein containing a little thrombosis becomes infected and inflamed, the resulting condition is called thrombophlebitis. It is characterised by a painful red line along the line of the affected vein.

Recommendations for massage

This is a local contraindication to massage. Light massage on the rest of the body is all right.

Deep vein thrombosis (DVT)

This is the serious condition mentioned previously. Risk factors are heavy smoking, pregnancy, major surgery, particularly to the knees, hips or pelvic area, and long-haul air travel. Unlike thrombophlebitis, DVT is difficult to diagnose. There may be pain behind the knees, or swollen calves, but there may be no symptoms.

Recommendations for massage

Since DVT is a potential killer, massage is totally contraindicated for three to six months after diagnosis, for practitioner protection. After that time period, the clot would be reduced by medication and the risk of an embolism minimal, but consult with the medical practitioner first about the advisability of massage and give gentle massage only. However, given the difficulty of diagnosis, it is advisable to be cautious about treating a person who has more than one risk factor in his case history. Examples might be a pregnant woman with painful legs, or a heavy smoker who has just got off a flight from Australia.

Arteriosclerosis

Arteriosclerosis refers to a general hardening, thickening and loss of elasticity of the walls of the arteries and a reduction in size of the hollow interior. Blood cannot be transported smoothly and quickly. This most common form of arterial disease can lead to heart attack or a stroke. Artherosclerosis is a form of arteriosclerosis, where fatty plaques develop on the walls, which could lead to clot formation. Risk factors are obesity, high blood pressure and diabetes.

Recommendations for massage

Consult with the medical practitioner first about the advisability of massage and give gentle, relaxing massage only.

DISORDERS OF THE HEART

Heart rate disorders/arrhythmias

In a normal healthy heart, the average rate is 60-100 per minute and varies according to physical exertion or emotional state. In an otherwise healthy person an unusually slow (bradycardia) rate is not a contraindication to massage. Tachycardia (high heart rate) is associated with other medical conditions, and the massage recommendations would be as for that condition.

Angina

This is a condition caused by inadequate blood supply to

the heart muscle. The coronary arteries bring blood to the heart muscle. When they become blocked, the condition called angina develops. Clots do not usually form in arteries; the coronary arteries are the one exception.

The symptoms of angina are cramp-like pains in the chest that are made worse by exercise or stress, and are relieved by rest. There is a particularly severe form of angina called unstable angina, and this can be a precursor to a heart attack.

Recommendations for massage

Relaxing massage is beneficial for people with angina because it can reduce stress. Keep the client warm, since cold can bring about an attack. Ask clients to bring their medication to the treatment in case of an attack. Massage for anyone with unstable angina should only be carried out after consulting the person's doctor.

Heart attack (or myocardial infarction)

If the function of the coronary arteries is badly impaired, part of the heart muscle doesn't get the blood supply it needs and dies. This is a heart attack. The symptoms are sudden and severe in the chest and the left arm, severe anxiety, nausea and restlessness. A heart attack can lead to sudden death.

Recommendations for massage

Because there is a very high risk of a reoccurrence in the

two to three months after the attack, massage is contraindicated for practitioner protection, and, after that, given with advice from the person's doctor. Use only gentle, relaxing massage.

Heart failure

If the heart is unable to perform its function as a pump properly, blood can back up in the lungs, causing pulmonary oedema, also called 'water on the lungs' or oedema in the ankles and legs. Heart failure can be caused by a number of different factors, including previous heart attacks or chronic high blood pressure.

Recommendations for massage

Consult with the medical practitioner first about the advisability of massage and give gentle, relaxing massage, to avoid stressing a weak heart. Avoid drainage techniques on areas of oedema.

Artificial pacemakers

These devices send out small electrical currents to stimulate heartbeat and are inserted under the pectoral muscles. If a client has a pacemaker, the pectoral region on the side of the pacemaker is a local contraindication. Offer supports under the chest for comfort when the client is lying on his front.

Chapter 9
Respiratory disorders

Disorders of parts of the respiratory tract are common, because of the direct connection with the environment and exposure to bacteria, viruses and pollutants. It is useful to remember that any medical term ending in 'itis' means 'inflammation of'; pharyngitis is inflammation of the pharynx, tonsillitis of the tonsils, bronchitis of the bronchioles, and so on. As a general rule, disorders of the upper part of the tract, from the nose to the larynx, are less serious than those affecting the lower part. Smokers have a much higher risk of developing respiratory disorders than non-smokers.

Many respiratory disorders are caused by bacteria or viruses, and are infectious in the early acute stages. Massage is contraindicated for two reasons: firstly, to avoid spread of disease to the massage therapist, and secondly, to avoid spread of infection around the body of the client. The decision to massage or not depends on the severity of the disorder. To catch a cold is very different from contracting pneumonia. It also depends on the stage of the illness. Many respiratory disorders, including pulmonary TB, pneumonia and bronchitis, are only infectious during the initial acute phase. In these cases, consult with the medical practitioner first to ascertain when the infectious period has passed.

When planning a treatment, remember that attention to the muscles involved in breathing can be very helpful for people with respiratory disorders. The muscles of unforced ordinary breathing are the intercostals and the diaphragm. The accessory muscles of breathing, those used in forced inhalation and exhalation, are the sternocleidomastoids, the scalenes and pectoralis minor. Coughing also puts unaccustomed pressure on the abdominal muscles. Chronic respiratory disorder results in tension in the whole upper body, and the postural muscles.

There are practical considerations for clients too. Breathing difficulties are often made worse by lying flat. If this is the case, it may be necessary to use supports to prop the client in a semi-sitting position, or in a side-lying position. Infections of the upper respiratory tract may make lying in a face hole or headrest uncomfortable. The quality of air in the treatment room is important for people with respiratory disorders. Make sure the room is well ventilated and free from chemicals (including essential oils in burners, air fresheners, or room sprays). Some respiratory disorders are aggravated by cold, so make sure the air is warm.

The common cold: recommendations for massage

The cold virus is infectious, and you are at risk if you

massage someone with a cold, but you are just as much at risk if you travel on public transport, go to the cinema or come into contact with lots of people.

Vigorous massage that speeds up circulation is inadvisable, but apart from that the decision is yours and your client's. Have tissues to hand, and be particularly careful with hygiene.

Influenza: recommendations for massage

This is contraindicated during the first few days, and probably someone with flu wouldn't want a massage anyway. After that time the same recommendations are the same as for a cold, but be aware that the flu virus hangs around in the body for several days after symptoms have gone, and the person is still infectious.

Sinusitis

This is inflammation of the air spaces in the head, causing pain and tenderness. The cause can be bacterial or viral, and sinusitis can also be an allergic reaction.

Recommendations for massage

If the cause is bacterial or viral, massage is contraindicated in the first few days, because the condition is infectious. There is no reason not to massage if the cause is allergic, but comfort is important. The person may not be comfortable lying horizontal for too long, or using a face hole or headrest.

Laryngitis

Inflammation of the larynx causes a sore throat and hoarseness or loss of voice.

Recommendations for massage

If not infectious, there is no reason not to massage.

Bronchitis

This refers to inflammation of the bronchi and/or bronchioles, resulting in over-production of mucous. Acute bronchitis often follows an upper respiratory infection. The inflammation causes over-secretion of mucous from the bronchi. Acute attacks often clear up after a few days. Chronic bronchitis refers to a state of chronic inflammation of the lower bronchi after years of acute bronchitis. This disease is associated with damp, pollution, dust and cigarette smoking, and the symptoms are coughing, production of phlegm, and breathing difficulties.

Recommendations for massage

Massage is contraindicated during the infectious phase of acute bronchitis. The person with chronic bronchitis can benefit from massage, particularly vibration and percussion on the back and chest to loosen phlegm and of the accessory muscles of breathing. Have tissues and a bowl available in case the client needs to cough up phlegm. Encourage the person to breathe deeply as part of the treatment.

Pneumonia

This condition means inflammation of the alveoli from bacterial or viral infection. Fluid accumulates in the alveoli. The symptoms are coughing, fever, and chest pain. For the first week or so, the person is quite unwell and probably wouldn't be coming for a massage treatment. Before the discovery of antibiotics, this was a serious, fatal disease. Pneumonia can still be a major cause of death, but nowadays usually in people who are already frail.

Recommendations for massage

Massage is contraindicated during the initial infectious phase of pneumonia. During the recovery phase, vibration and percussion techniques on the back and chest are helpful to move fluid. Massage of the accessory muscles of breathing and the postural muscles of the back helps. If the person has been in bed for some time, massage the lower limbs and use passive joint manipulations to help circulation. Lying horizontal for too long may be uncomfortable, so prop the person up with pillows.

Emphysema

Bronchitis can develop into emphysema. The walls of the alveoli are destroyed and breathing becomes very difficult.

Recommendations for massage

Calming relaxation massage with attention to the accessory muscles of breathing and the whole back, chest and neck area is beneficial. The person may not be able to lie down, so prop up with pillows or consider massaging in a chair.

Asthma

Asthma is a common condition that affects one in seven people. The muscles surrounding the bronchioles in the lungs constrict, preventing easy passage of air though the tubes. Breathing in increases the space in the lungs and eases the problem, but breathing out creates compression in the lungs that increases the constriction. Asthmatics have trouble breathing out, and their breath often sounds wheezy. The shoulder muscles may be used to help force air out of the lungs during an attack. The normal process of expelling mucous from the tubes is hampered by the constriction. The resulting build-up of mucous gives rise to secondary complications. An asthmatic attack can be very frightening for the sufferer.

Recommendations for massage

General relaxation massage is beneficial for asthma sufferers. Some asthmatics are sensitive to flower pollen, animal hair or strong scents. Ask about possible allergens that can trigger an attack, and make sure that you have none in the treatment room.

Check that the person has an inhaler or medication present in the event of an attack. Negotiate a comfortable position; some asthmatics may feel more comfortable lying on their side. Pay attention to the accessory muscles of breathing and to the whole neck and shoulder area.

Pleurisy

Inflammation of the pleura, the lining around the lungs and inside the ribcage, causes a sharp stabbing pain when breathing.

Recommendations for massage

If the cause is bacterial, massage is contraindicated in the acute stages. After that, relaxation massage, with attention to the accessory muscles of breathing and to the back neck and shoulders, is helpful.

Lung cancer

This is the commonest form of cancer in men. There may be two to three years between the development of cancer and the appearance of any symptoms.

Recommendations for massage

Relaxation massage is beneficial to help relieve stress with all forms of cancer, but take the current level vitality of the person into account when deciding on the length of treatment, pressure of strokes and kinds of techniques used. Never massage directly over any tumour or site of cancer, or areas currently receiving radiotherapy.

Observe the usual contraindications about broken skin, infections, recent scar tissue, and cardiovascular complications. Be aware that chemotherapy and radiotherapy can cause thin skin. (See also 'massage and cancer'.)

Tuberculosis (TB)

This bacterial infection once killed hundreds of people, and is on the increase again amongst the elderly, immigrant populations, the homeless and those who are HIV positive. Many people carry the bacteria that cause TB without ever developing the disease. The most common form is pulmonary TB, but it can affect other tissues in the body. Inhaling the bacteria in droplets from coughs and sneezes in the air can transmit the disease. Symptoms are general malaise, weight loss, coughing and night sweats.

Recommendations for massage

Pulmonary tuberculosis is not generally infectious two to four weeks after the start of treatment with medication. Massage is contraindicated until this stage, so consult with the medical practitioner first about the advisability of massage. Take the person's level of vitality into account.

Chapter 10
Pain and nociception

Pain

All pathology could be said to involve the nervous system since pain is the body's way of signalling that all is not well. One of the functions of the nerves and neurochemicals, together with the immune system, is to inform the whole body about attack or threat to the tissues from external trauma, internal imbalance, or the presence of harmful bacteria or viruses. Whether the problem is a boil (the integumentary system), a sprain (musculoskeltal system), or menstrual cramps (reproductive system), we know about it because sensory nerve receptors are firing away, sending their messages to the brain.

Nociception

Nociception is the term that describes the response of the nervous system to real or potential damage to the tissues. Nociceptive receptors respond to extreme temperature, pressure, light and sound, and to irritants released from damaged cells, and transmit this information to the spinal cord and then the brain. Pain is an unpleasant sensory and emotional response associated with actual or potential tissue damage, or the perception of such tissue damage. There are more than 70 words in English to describe pain. Pain is a subjective experience, varying from person to person. Pain and nociception are not the same thing. There is no clear or consistent correspondence between the experience of pain and tissue damage. Here are two extreme examples. When a person is in real danger, he is able to flee from the source with a broken leg and only on reaching safety will he begin to experience any pain. There is real tissue damage but no awareness of pain. On the other hand, many amputees describe discomfort or pain in their limbs that no longer exist. Pain is experienced in the absence of tissue damage. This is called the 'phantom limb' phenomenon.

Massage and pain

One of the consistent research findings about the benefits of massage is that touch alleviates the perception of pain. Light pressure, vibration and touch on the skin activate certain sensory nerves, which then block the signals from tissue damage from being transmitted to the brain via other nerves. Sensations arising from touch to the skin or non-painful manipulation of soft tissue arrive at the brain before pain sensations, and help to displace the awareness of pain.

Any activity that eases contraction in muscles that have 'splinted' around chronic pain, such as progressive muscle relaxation, yoga or biofeedback, as well as massage, reduces secondary causes of pain.

Chapter 11
Nervous system disorders

As well as being the system that signals the presence of pain, there are disorders that specifically affect or arise in the tissues of the central nervous system or peripheral nerves, or that affect the balance of neurochemicals in the body.

Many nervous system disorders have complicated or unknown origin, but sometimes the causes are clearly due to infection, trauma or degeneration. Some affect motor nerves and therefore the functioning of skeletal and visceral muscle. Some affect sensory nerves and the ability to detect touch, pressure, pain and proprioception (other information about the body, including muscle tension, balance and position in space), or the functioning of the other special senses. And some disorders affect mental functioning and mood.

In Chapters 11 to 13 we will consider those that affect motor and sensory nerve function and that require particular physical considerations when it comes to planning the massage treatment. In Chapters 14 and 15, we will think about how to work with people who are experiencing mood disorders or mental health problems.

Many nervous system disorders cause serious problems for the individual affected. Acute conditions, such as a stroke or meningitis, can be fatal, but the person may recover with little or no after-effects. Conditions like multiple sclerosis and Parkinson's disease are chronic and degenerative, with ongoing symptoms that may vary from time to time. And other conditions arise from a congenital problem, injury or infection that has long past but has left a permanent mark on the body. Polio, spina bifida and spinal cord injury come into this category.

CONDITIONS THAT AFFECT THE PERIPHERAL NERVES

Neuralgia, neuropathy and neuritis

These terms tend to be muddled in common usage. They all refer to the peripheral nerves and may be associated with one of the chronic conditions described later, but can also be temporary phenomena. Inflammation of a peripheral nerve is neuritis ('neur' – nerve and 'itis' – inflammation) and any other disorder, apart from inflammation, is called neuropathy ('neuro' – nerve and 'pathy' – disorder). The pain arising from neuritis or neuropathy is called neuralgia. Peripheral neuropathy is a condition associated with long-term diabetes, alcoholism, circulation disorders and vitamin B deficiency, but it can also arise from pressure on a nerve when it presses against surrounding soft tissue, or is trapped against hard tissue, such as bone or cartilage. The symptoms range from pins and needles, and tingling, to pain, numbness along the path of the nerve, and, if it's a motor nerve that's affected, loss of function in the muscle that the nerve innervates.

Recommendations for massage

Treatment decisions depend on the individual, and on other medical complications that need taking into account. Muscles contract protectively around pain, so massage to relieve muscle tension is beneficial. However, avoid deep pressure where there is loss of sensation, and avoid areas of hypersensitivity.

Carpal tunnel syndrome

The causes of this include repetitive strain injury, but it is also associated with other conditions, such as diabetes or rheumatoid arthritis. The tendon sheath to the wrist and finger muscles becomes inflamed, causing compression of the median nerve.

Recommendations for massage

Carpal tunnel syndrome is an occupational hazard for massage therapists, so make sure you massage your own hands and forearms regularly, and use neck, shoulder and wrist mobilisation and stretching exercises. With clients, avoid massage directly on the wrist if there is pain or inflammation, otherwise use transverse friction. Massage the rest of the arms, neck and shoulders thoroughly, and use joint mobilisation techniques on the shoulder, elbow and wrist.

Sciatica

A very common condition, sciatica is pain and numbness along the sciatic nerve, most often felt in the buttocks and thighs. There may be loss of sensation and function in the leg muscles. It may be caused by compression or by damage from injury. Compression at the point of exit from the spinal cord can be caused by a herniated disc or a fractured vertebra. Compression further along can be caused by tension in the pirifomis muscle.

Recommendations for massage

The cause of the problem, if known, should be taken into account. The general aims are to stimulate circulation in the muscles affected, and assist muscles to relax to avoid spasm. If there is loss of sensation, avoid deep pressure, also to be avoided along the sciatic nerve path itself. Use joint mobilisations of the knee, ankle and toes, and massage compensating muscles in the lower back and other leg thoroughly.

Bell's palsy

The facial nerve is unusual in that it carries only motor nerve fibres. Damage to the facial nerve results in paralysis of some of the facial muscles on one side of the head, but with no loss of sensation. There is difficulty eating, speaking and closing the eye on the affected side. This is called Bell's palsy. Onset is usually very sudden, but recovery is often quick as well, depending on the underlying cause.

Recommendations for massage

Consult with the medical practitioner first about the

advisability of massage, in case the underlying cause is a contraindication. If not, massage of the facial muscles, head and neck is definitely beneficial. It may be helpful to massage the face in two halves, starting with the unaffected side.

Trigeminal neuralgia

This is another condition that affects a facial nerve, but unlike Bell's palsy, there is excruciating pain along the nerve pathway, on one or both sides of the face. The pain is not consistent but can be easily triggered. The cause is unknown. Trigeminal neuralgia is a chronic condition that can be very hard to live with.

Recommendations for massage

People with this condition may not want to be touched anywhere on the face or head, but general relaxation massage of the rest of the body is beneficial. Negotiate with the client about face and head contact, and about whether she can tolerate lying on her front, or with her face in a headrest.

Shingles

The herpes zoster virus, which is responsible for chicken pox in children, can be reactivated in adults. Toxins are released, which cause inflammation of the sensory nerves in the intercostal area. Symptoms are pain and a blistery rash. There may also be blisters on the face, following the trigeminal nerve pathway. This condition is a local contraindication to massage, but the person may feel too unwell to be massaged.

CONDITIONS THAT AFFECT THE CENTRAL NERVOUS SYSTEM

Headaches and migraine

Massage is generally beneficial for these commonplace conditions, with two exceptions. Do not massage if someone has a sudden-onset, severe headache for no apparent reason, but suggest they get medical help because this could be the precursor to something serious. And it is not advisable to massage someone during a migraine attack, although they probably wouldn't want it! The type of headache more commonly found in massage clients is stress-related, and this type usually develops from tension in the skull and facial muscles. Massage of these areas, as well as the neck and shoulders, is beneficial.

Migraines are a particular form of headache and affect about 10 per cent of people. Constriction of the blood vessels around the temples may contribute to the cause, and so may stress. Daily self-massage of the temporalis and masseter muscles can play an important part in a treatment programme, so teach your client how to do this. Regular professional massage can help to reduce stress levels.

Epilepsy

An epileptic fit, or seizure, is caused by abnormal electrical activity in the brain. There are different types of seizure, ranging from momentary lapses in attention with tingling sensations in the limbs, to the 'grand mal', or major fit, where the person loses consciousness for a few minutes. Epileptics often have a warning sign, known as an aura, of an impending fit. Except in severe cases, fitting is usually controlled by medication.

Recommendations for massage

Do not attempt to massage someone who is having a fit; otherwise, massage is not contraindicated. Essential oils may trigger a seizure, so avoid their use. Some practitioners who work with energy have reported that working with energy around the head area has brought on epileptic fits, so it may be advisable for those who intentionally work with energy during massage to avoid input to the head area.

If a client has an aura and senses an impending seizure, put him in the recovery position on the ground, well away from walls or hard objects. Put a small rolled towel in his mouth to prevent him biting his tongue, but do not force the jaw open if it is clenched. After the seizure, the body may be too sore to massage.

Stroke (cerebrovascular accident, CVA)

If the blood supply to the brain is affected, either by a clot (thrombosis) that cuts off the supply to the tissues or by a blood vessel bursting and leaking into the tissue, part of the brain tissue is damaged. Depending on the part involved, this may result in loss of speech, movement, sensation, thinking ability, or sphincter control. Strokes can be fatal.

Recommendations for massage

There is a very high risk of a second stroke occurring within one month of the first, so do not massage someone at all during this period, for your own protection. There is a lower risk of a stroke occurring up to six months after the first, and, during this period, it is advisable to notify the client's doctor and ask if there are any reasons not to massage. During the rehabilitation period, massage can assist physiotherapy by stretching contracted muscles and facilitating joint mobility, as well as being psychologically supportive to the stroke patient. There may well be other cardiovascular problems that you need to take into account when planning a treatment. Avoid any techniques that stimulate the circulation.

Transient ischaemic attack (TIA)

A TIA is a mini-stroke lasting a few minutes from which the person recovers with no or little damage. TIAs are caused by clots in the arteries of the neck, which temporarily cut off blood supply to the brain.

Recommendations for massage

Since there is a high risk of further TIAs, medical advice should be sought before massage is given.

Meningitis

Meningitis is inflammation of the meninges, which are the connective tissue coverings of the brain and spinal cord.

Symptoms include fever, severe headache, and a stiff neck. In the acute stage, this condition is a total contraindication and requires hospital treatment. There is no reason to prevent someone who has recovered from meningitis from having massage.

A herniated or 'slipped' disc

A herniated disc refers to compression of a nerve root arising when a vertebral disc ruptures and part of the contents is displaced on to the spinal nerve. It most commonly affects L4/5 or the lumbar-sacral joint. People sometimes refer to any sharp back pain as a slipped disc, but an actual slipped disc is very painful and debilitating. It can cause sciatica.

Recommendations for massage

If the pain in the spinal muscles near the site is on one side only, this is more likely to be a trapped nerve, which massage may ease. If the pain is on both sides of the spine, it is more likely to be a slipped disc, in which case refer the client to an osteopath, chiropractor or physiotherapist. When the most acute stage has subsided, gentle massage, sensitively applied, may help to relieve pain from associated muscle spasms.

Spinal cord injury

Symptoms of spinal cord injury depend on the site of the damage. Generally speaking, there will be impairment of motor and sensory functions below the injury, although some motor reflexes that are independent of brain control remain intact. There may be spasticity and loss of tone in the muscles, or muscles that spasm to touch and are floppy. A person with spinal cord injury has to come to terms with life-changing impairment, and if the injury is recent, the person's mental and emotional state needs to be taken into account.

Recommendations for massage

Massage is beneficial for physical reasons and also for general well-being. Negotiate with the client about position, use of supports, pressure of strokes used and when moving joints, both as part of the treatment and when helping the person into position. Maintaining joint flexibility and circulation to muscles is important. Use gentle, rhythmic, repetitive strokes. Muscles that spasm to touch respond to this type of contact. If there is also sensory loss, take great care with pressure and joint movements since the client will not be able to give accurate feedback about what you are doing. Wheelchair users are susceptible to pressure sores, and these areas should be avoided. Non-ambulant people also have thin skin on the soles of the feet, so avoid pressure or friction strokes here. See also the section on other considerations when working with people who are physically vulnerable.

Spina bifida

This condition is a congenital defect in the vertebrae, usually in the lumbar spine. The bone fails to form properly over the spinal cord, leaving parts exposed. In the more common, mild form, there may be no symptoms or some weakness in the legs. In the severe form, there is paralysis and impairment of bladder function.

Recommendations for massage

Mild spina bifida is a local contraindication to massage in the lumbar sacral area of the back. For severe cases, see recommendations for spinal cord injury.

Poliomyelitis

Since the advent of vaccination for polio in 1957 this condition has disappeared in the UK, although there are people who were affected before this date or were born in countries where the vaccine is not available. The polio virus affects motor neurons in the spinal cord and can result in paralysis. The muscles become floppy and wasted, and the antagonists become over-stretched to compensate.

Recommendations for massage

All the recommendations for spinal cord injuries apply.

Parkinson's disease

This degenerative disorder affects voluntary movements and is characterised by muscle rigidity and sluggishness, and tremors arising from uncontrollable muscle twitching. If the speech muscles are affected, communication may become difficult. Stress can make tremors worse. Parkinson's disease is associated with an imbalance of neurochemicals in the brain, particularly dopamine.

Recommendations for massage

Massage may be beneficial as a means of stimulating circulation, bringing nutrients to the muscles and removing wastes. If there is also sensory loss, take great care with pressure and joint movements since the client will not be able to give accurate feedback about what you are doing. Assist the client into position for treatment if he suffers poor muscle control or tremors. With increasing stiffness, a client with Parkinson's disease may not be able to get on and off a treatment couch, and you may want to massage in a chair or on the floor.

Treatment decisions need to take into account the person's condition on that day, as well as other conditions that may be present, such as thin skin.

Multiple sclerosis (MS)

Degeneration of the myelin sheath around the axons in the CNS results in the condition known as multiple sclerosis. The symptoms depend on the part of the brain affected, and include loss of vision, weakness and numbness in the legs. A person with MS may have periods of remission from symptoms, sometimes for years at a time.

Recommendations for massage

The recommendations for spinal cord injuries apply, but also remember that people with MS get tired very easily, so avoid working for too long a period, or using techniques that could deplete the body.

Cerebral palsy

There are a number of conditions that result from damage to the brain during or soon after birth. There is always some lack of muscle control, and may be communication or learning difficulties. Hemiplegia refers to paralysis on one side of the body only, quadraplegia to paralysis of all four limbs, and paraplegia to the lower half of the body.

Recommendations for massage

These are the same as for spinal cord injuries. If the person finds it hard to communicate, suggest using an advocate who understands the person well.

Chapter 12
Massage for the physically vulnerable

The umbrella term 'physically vulnerable' includes people with physical impairment (temporary, like a fractured femur in a plaster cast, or permanent, like a limb affected by polio) and/or disability (paralysis from birth injury or accident), and frailty arising from a debilitating illness (chronic fatigue syndrome), or from extreme age. If you have ever broken an arm or leg, or put one hand out of action by cutting a finger, if you can remember the complete lethargy that follows a bout of flu, then you have a slight idea of what it is like to live with physical vulnerability. For many people who are physically vulnerable, life is like that all the time. Imagine the frustration, shame or embarrassment of being slower, or less able than others, or what it must be like to depend on carers for help with dressing or feeding or walking. Imagine what it must feel like to look unusual, or be stared at, to feel different from others and afraid of being judged. Imagine how it feels living with a condition that you know will deteriorate and eventually be the cause of your death. We need to be sensitive to the emotional and psychological aspects of living with a physical impairment. On the one hand, we can't relate to the person as if he were able-bodied; on the other hand, we can't assume that we know what it's like to live in his body. Just because he is slower or needs assistance, he is not a child – don't infantilise! We also need to be aware of our own reaction to, and feelings about, physical impairment.

People who have needed a lot of medical attention, such as operations, periods in hospital, nursing care, or physiotherapy, will have had considerable experience of being touched in a particular way. Without wanting to imply that all health care professionals are lacking in sensitivity, there is a way that patients can be treated as if they were just bodies, and faulty bodies at that. There may be little choice about being touched, or refusing painful or uncomfortable touch. It may be helpful to explain that massage is not meant to be uncomfortable and that the person can make choices about how she is touched and where.

General care

If you are working in a private practice or a salon or health centre, in other words any environment that is not specifically designed to cater for the needs of physically vulnerable people, then a rough assessment of need in relation to the facilities available should be made prior to the first attendance. It's no use to a wheelchair user to arrive for a massage and find that the treatment room is on the fourth floor! Allow more time for the initial consultation and for dressing and undressing. Be prepared to adapt how you work and negotiate with your client about where would be most comfortable to be massaged – in a chair or on the couch – and how to position and support her body. Remember that if there is sensory loss, she may not be able to give accurate feedback. If she has equipment with her, like a wheelchair, braces, breathing apparatus or even walking stick, ask where she would like them to be during the treatment. If she has incontinence problems, be sensitive to potential embarrassment, and straightforward about discussing practical possibilities.

The massage treatment

Take any associated medical conditions into account when planning the treatment. Seek active consent from your client, and check pressure, comfort, and speed as you go along. Be sensitive to non-verbal signs of discomfort and of pleasure. People who are non-ambulant have thinner skin on the soles of their feet – be gentle here. Avoid pressure sores, but be aware too that lifting and gently massaging limbs can help prevent such sores. If your client uses her hands or feet for support, do not use oil on them, or ensure that you remove oil at the end of the massage.

Chapter 13
Sensory disorders

Visual impairment

Under this heading come long and short sight, both of which can be corrected by wearing glasses or contact lenses, and the more disabling visual impairments that can lead to complete blindness. However, a person who is registered blind may have some sight. Cataracts are common in elderly people and are treated with a lens replacement operation. Glaucoma refers to damage to the optic nerve, usually from an increase in pressure in the eyeball. There are a number of visual disorders arising from long-term diabetes.

Considerations for massage

There is no reason not to massage anyone with a visual impairment, and relaxation massage would probably be beneficial if living with the impairment causes stress or anxiety. The muscles around the eyes may benefit from massage, with consent from the client, but avoid direct pressure on the eyeballs. With diabetic visual problems, observe other appropriate recommendations for massage. Practical issues include making provision for a guide dog, if necessary, keeping the layout of the room the same or informing the client if items have been changed, and avoiding moving the client's possessions. Ask if he would prefer to remove contact lenses or glasses, and with the latter, if he would like them close by during the treatment. If someone cannot see what you are doing, or what you want him to do, talk it through clearly. Maybe talk about what you are doing during the massage, especially on a first visit. Ask him how much assistance he would like moving around the room and getting on and off the couch.

Hearing impairment

Deafness can be innate or acquired, and can vary from a mild loss, usually difficulty hearing conversation in noisy places, to profound loss, when no sound is intelligible. Some hearing-impaired people use British Sign Language to communicate, and some wear hearing aids, and most lip read. The speech of a hearing impaired person may be hard to follow if she was born deaf or became deaf before she learned to speak.

Considerations for massage

At all times, make sure your face is visible so that the person can lip read easily. Keep your face in the light, don't cover your mouth with your hand, and speak clearly. If the person has a 'good' ear, position yourself to speak to that side. Ask if your client wants to remove her aids during the treatment, and then remember that she won't be able to hear you at all. Negotiate pre-arranged signs for 'turn over now' or for your client to use to signal discomfort.

Tinnitus

Tinnitus refers to sounds like buzzing, whistling or roaring in one or both ears. It can come and go, and has no known cause. There may or may not be hearing loss as well. Some tinnitus sufferers wear an aid that makes white noise to mask the sounds.

Considerations for massage

Relaxation massage is beneficial, tinnitus being a stressful condition to live with. However, since it often seems worse at night, when there is little other external noise to distract from it, it may help the client to offer background music.

Chapter 14

Communication and cognitive disorders

There are groups of people who have some aspect of nervous system dysfunction that affects cognitive or emotional functioning. If the massage therapist is working with a special needs group in a residential setting, day-care centre or hospital, she has access to medical information, support and, hopefully, training that will enable her to work effectively with that group. The guidelines below are intended for the special needs of clients we might encounter in everyday practice – and to provoke thought about good practice in general.

The idea that a treatment is contraindicated or indicated comes from the medical model and usually applies to the physical body. When talking about pathology and massage for the other systems of the body, the main focus is on different medical conditions and whether massage is beneficial or not, and, if it is, then how to massage. Other aspects of the massage treatment that are taken for granted as normal good practice are the relationship between the therapist and client, and the environment in which the massage takes place.

Working with people with special needs regarding communication or emotional vulnerability, the focus widens to include consideration of the relationship and the environment as part of the 'how to' aspect of planning a massage treatment. The mental and emotional states of being of our clients have to be taken into account as much as their physical bodies.

Cognitive impairment: dyslexia

People who have dyslexia have difficulty recognising, writing or remembering written symbols – letters, words or numbers.

Recommendations for massage

There is no reason not to massage someone who has dyslexia. If you ask clients to fill in written medical histories or consent forms as part of your practice, remember that a dyslexic client may not be able to do this easily.

Learning impairment

People with learning impairment, sometimes referred to as 'learning difficulty', have, as the name suggests, more difficulty learning than other people. This condition ranges for mild to severe, may be present at birth or may develop after a childhood illness. It includes people with Down's syndrome and those with autistic spectrum disorder, who have particular difficulty with interpersonal relating.

Recommendations for massage

There is a higher incidence of epilepsy associated with learning impairment. If present, observe the appropriate precautions. People with Down's syndrome often have poor muscle tone and hypermobile joints. Take care with joint manipulations and aim to increase muscle tone. People with learning difficulty also have some degree of communication impairment; see the guidelines in the following section.

Dementia

A group of conditions, the commonest being Alzheimer's disease, dementia involves progressive loss of memory, perception and speech.

Recommendations for massage

Relaxation massage is helpful if the person is not over-anxious. Motor function is affected as the condition progresses, and massage can help with muscle function and joint flexibility. Informed consent from a carer is needed, together with a full case history to take into account any other complications. See the guidelines in the following section for communication difficulties.

Communication difficulty

Communication involves the ability to understand language and the ability to produce meaningful speech. A person with a learning difficulty may be affected in both areas, but a person who has lost the use of his muscles of speech production, which can happen after a stroke, with MS or Parkinson's disease, may have perfect comprehension. Someone with dementia may have both abilities but her short-term memory loss means she can't remember what has just been said.

Recommendations for massage

Taking into account any other medical conditions that may be present, there is no reason not to massage someone with a communication difficulty, but the relational aspects of the whole treatment need special consideration. The client may not be able to understand you, and/or you may not be able to understand the client. He may be accompanied by a family member, carer or advocate, to speak for him, in which case you need to be sensitive to issues of confidentiality, and to include the client as much as possible in the consultation, to avoid a 'Does he take sugar?' situation.

Establish an appropriate method of communication. Face the client and make use of facial expression and gesture, and use simple language if he has a comprehension difficulty. This would be inappropriate and infantilising in a person with good understanding! If the client has trouble speaking clearly, allow time, ask for clarification and repeat what's been said to check if you've got it right. Don't pretend to understand if you don't, and use writing, if appropriate.

Explain as clearly as you can what will happen. If your

client has a history of extensive medical treatment or currently lives in an institution, he may not be used to making choices about his treatment, so try to establish that you expect him to do this and be sensitive to what he seems to want. If he has a history of painful or invasive treatments, he may be anxious about having massage, so go slowly. For example, consider only massaging hands or feet on an initial visit. It may help to establish a simple signal, like raising a hand, for the client to use for 'this is not okay', so that she has a simple way to let you know during the treatment if she's uncomfortable. Be sensitive to changes in autonomic nervous system responses, and other non-verbal cues, in the client while you are working. Allow more time for aftercare as well as the initial consultation.

Chapter 15
Emotional vulnerability

Post-traumatic stress

When someone is exposed to a traumatic situation (a train crash, rape, witnessing a violent attack) her sympathetic nervous system goes into high arousal. If the effects are not discharged, this arousal gets locked into the system, causing post-traumatic stress. The symptoms are the same as for everyday stress but persist in the absence of current triggers, causing sleep and appetite disturbance, problems with attention and memory, and ongoing anxiety and distress.

Many people experience some degree of post-traumatic stress, sometimes without being aware of the initial trigger. Survivors of sexual, physical or emotional abuse, refugees, and victims of violence are all people at risk of post-traumatic stress.

Recommendations for massage

Relaxation massage is helpful to establish parasympathetic

activity in the nervous system, but bear in mind that there may be many aspects of the massage situation that could act as triggers for arousal in someone suffering from post-traumatic stress. Be sensitive to signs of sympathetic nervous system arousal in your client through the initial consultation and treatment. Issues of trust and safety are very important, and it helps the client if you are very clear about your boundaries and maintain a professional relationship. Be clear about time and money as well. Negotiate with your client about the treatment and discuss options. Be explicit about what you will do and stick to it!

People who are emotionally vulnerable may find it hard to talk about their bodies or their feelings, and a simple question like "What sort of massage would you like?" may create anxiety because the client just doesn't know. It may help to ask fairly concrete questions in the initial interview. "Would you like to feel relaxed or alert after the massage?" "Which part of your body is uncomfortable?"

It may help to establish a prearranged signal for 'stop now' or 'that's enough' and practise it before you begin the massage so your client can trust that you will use it. Consider using a running commentary as you massage. "I'm going to rest my hands here for a moment, and then I'll uncover your back and start to oil your skin." Keep comments neutral. Forget any assumptions you have that massage only works if the client is silent! She may also want to keep her eyes open. Be flexible. The most important thing is her feeling of safety.

Survivors of sexual or physical abuse may have difficulty

recognising the difference between sexual and non-sexual touch, or between nurturing and abusive touch. All the suggestions for working with someone with post-traumatic stress apply, and it can be helpful, if the client becomes anxious during the treatment, to actually state that you are not going to hit her, touch her inappropriately or hurt her. Be sensitive and use your discretion. Survivors may also have difficulties with the idea of lying down or removing clothes. Be prepared to be flexible.

Eating disorders

Compulsive eating, anorexia (refusal to eat) and bulimia (bingeing then vomiting) are all conditions that involve negative or distorted body image and low self-worth. Severe anorexia nervosa can be fatal and may require hospital treatment. Bulimia poses less of a serious risk to physical health unless it is a part of an anorexic condition.

Recommendations for massage

Relaxation massage can help a person with an eating disorder feel more positive about herself and her body. Be careful to keep comments about her body neutral. A person with advanced anorexia is very frail, with wasted muscles and thin skin, so use gentle massage only.

Chemical dependency

The whole subject of chemical dependency and abuse is loaded with questions and value judgements. At what point does alcohol use stop being social drinking and become alcoholism? Why is addiction to a legal substance like caffeine more acceptable than addiction to cocaine? When does use of a substance become abuse? Excessive consumption of any substance can be injurious to health, and massage therapists are concerned with the general well-being of our clients. However, we have to be careful not to assume a client has a substance problem if he hasn't indicated as much. We must be aware of our own feelings about the issue and walk a fine line between offering support and telling a client what we think he should do.

Recommendations for massage

If a client arrives for a massage under the influence of alcohol or non-prescribed drugs, massage is contraindicated, to protect the practitioner as well as the client. Serious long-term alcohol or drug use causes many different health problems, which must be taken into account when planning a massage. People in recovery from chemical dependency can benefit a lot from massage, as a non-chemical means of feeling good about themselves.

Panic and anxiety attacks

Anxiety is a common feeling, sometimes linked to a particular event, such as visiting the dentist or being on time for an appointment, but sometimes a person can feel anxious for no particular reason. A panic attack is an extreme form of anxiety, which comes on suddenly (hence the term 'attack') and is shockingly frightening. The person often feels as if he is about to die or go crazy. Having one panic attack can lead to anxiety about further attacks.

Recommendations for massage

Anxiety and panic attacks both result from sympathetic nervous system arousal, so relaxation massage is indicated here. Some people find it very helpful to have the physiology of the stress response explained to them, because it gives an ordinary context to an extraordinary experience. Advice and exercises to help the client breathe properly are very beneficial.

Depression

There are many kinds and degrees of depression, ranging from 'having a down day' to a severe illness that might need hospital treatment. Some depressions have an organic cause and others are triggered by external events. Depression can be part of a normal process of adjustment or can be a serious medical condition.

Recommendations for massage

Massage is indicated for a depressed person as a way of helping him feel better about himself. There is also evidence linking depression with dysfunction of the hypothalamus/pituitary/adrenal axis, so relaxation massage will help to re-establish the normal working of the autonomic nervous system.

What to do if a client starts crying

Emotional release can be a normal outcome from massage – you haven't done anything wrong! If you notice tears leaking or trickling out of the eyes, with little noticeable change in breathing, ask if the client is okay or if they would like a tissue. Let your client know that you've noticed, but keep your response light and neutral. You don't have to stop massaging. If your client begins to sob or cry noisily, tell her you're going to stop the massage for a while, and ask her to curl on her side. This is easier for breathing and usually feels safer. Offer tissues. Sit with her, with a hand on her arm or hand until she quietens. You don't have to do anything. She may want to talk about it, and, if so, all you have to do is listen. You don't have to make it all right – that isn't your job.

When the tears have subsided, ask her whether she'd like to continue the massage or stop. Offer water. Ascertain, if you don't already know, whether she has professional help or someone to talk to. If appropriate, offer a referral to a counselling or psychotherapy agency.

Chapter 16
Immune disorders

The immune system has two functional aspects, one that we are born with, and one that develops after birth. The innate aspect gets triggered automatically by any sort of foreign matter, or antigen, entering the body, or by tissue damage. Inflammation is an example of this aspect of the body's defence mechanisms. Allergies are examples of the body's natural defence mechanisms working overtime.

The other aspect, called acquired immunity, is more specific, only reacting to foreign matter that it has already been exposed to and has learned to recognise. If you had any of the common childhood diseases, such as chicken pox, or have been vaccinated against them, your immune system has acquired an immunity to these diseases.

Auto-immune diseases, cancer, and HIV/AIDS are examples of failures of acquired immunity. The body reacts to its own tissues as if they were foreign material. These diseases are poorly understood. They include vitiligo (the skin), multiple sclerosis (the nerves), myasthenia gravis (the muscles) and rheumatoid arthritis.

Inflammation

The inflammatory response is one of the body's innate defence mechanisms. It is a non-specific response to tissue injury, which aims to wall off the affected area from the surrounding tissue, remove disease-causing organisms, and remove dead tissue and replace it with new tissue or scar formation. It lasts from a few hours to a few days. The symptoms are redness (if near the surface of the body) from localised vasodilation, which also, together with fluid leakage from capillaries, causes swelling, heat and pain, resulting from the pressure on sensory nerves. Inflammation in muscle or joints may result in loss of function.

Recommendations for massage

Inflammation is always a local contraindication to massage.

Allergies

When the immune system over-reacts to harmless antigens and treats them as dangerous invaders, allergic symptoms are produced. Common allergies are hay fever, allergic asthma and skin rashes, including eczema. Some people have allergic reactions to foods, such as shellfish, eggs, milk, and strawberries.

Recommendations for massage

Respect a person's allergies by avoiding use of essential oils in massage oil or aromatherapy burners, by using vegetable rather than nut-based carrier oils, and by not using perfumed soaps, deodorants or body lotions yourself. If a client's skin becomes red, hot or itchy during a massage, it may be an allergic reaction to the oil or cream being used. Wipe the oil off the area and discuss continuing the massage through the towel, without oil.

Anaphylactic shock

A severe allergic response can cause a sudden drop in blood pressure, breathing difficulties and even death. This is called anaphylactic shock. Someone who has experienced this condition may carry a syringe of adrenaline with them.

Recommendations for massage

If anaphylactic shock is mentioned in the case history, check whether the client has medication with her. If a client goes into shock, this is a medical emergency and you should call an ambulance immediately.

Chronic fatigue syndrome

The cause of chronic fatigue syndrome is unknown. The symptoms are extreme fatigue over a long period that isn't resolved by rest and sleep. Normal activity becomes impaired, the sufferer is irritable and depressed, and experiences muscle/joint pain and weakness, and sleep problems.

Recommendations for massage

Gentle whole-body massage is beneficial for people with

this disorder because it can help restore parasympathetic activity and relaxation, it can relieve muscle and joint pain, and can stimulate sluggish circulation in the muscles. The symptoms can vary, for any individual, on a daily basis, so it is important, with a regular client, to ask about his state of health on each visit and to tailor the treatment accordingly.

Cancer

No one really understands the process that causes some cells to proliferate too rapidly, or to develop abnormal forms. Usually, the immune system deals with these cells by destroying them, but sometimes this process fails and the cells grow out of control and large masses of abnormal tissue develop. These are called tumours, and there are two kinds.

Benign tumours are not harmful, unless they are exerting pressure on other internal organs. Malignant tumours are the ones commonly called cancers, and they can spread rapidly, invading other types of tissues. The most common cancers in men are of the lung, colon, prostate and pancreas, and in women, of the lung, colon, uterus and breast.

Recommendations for massage

Although it is true that some cancers are spread through the lymphatic system, and that massage may affect the flow of lymph, there is no evidence that massage can spread cancer cells. The National Guidelines for the use of Complementary Therapies in Supportive and Palliative Care, published by the Foundation for Integrated Health in May 2003, state that massage is an acceptable intervention for people with cancer. (Bristol Cancer Help Centre, 2003. Massage policy for people with cancer.) Soothing, relaxing massage is generally beneficial for people with cancer. Massage can provide a valuable source of comfort and relief from emotional stress. It is a source of caring touch for a person experiencing intensive medical treatment. It may help to relieve pain on a temporary basis, and it may help with sleeping difficulties, minor digestive problems, and muscular stiffness.

Decisions about the length, type and which parts of the body to massage depend on the type of cancer, how far advanced it is, the kind of medical treatments the person is having, and the client's general health and vitality at the time of the session. However, observe the following recommendations.

❶ If the client is receiving treatment, ask permission to consult his medical practitioner about the advisability of massage. If the client has recovered from, or is in remission from, cancer, there is no reason not to massage.
❷ Never massage directly over any tumour or site of cancer, or undiagnosed lumps or swellings.
❸ Avoid techniques that stimulate the circulation, unless you are trained in manual lymphatic drainage, and any deep tissue work.
❹ Radiotherapy is a treatment that uses radiation into the body to shrink tumours. The site of radiation may be tender – the skin may become thin, or even burnt. This area is a local contraindication to massage.

❺ Chemotherapy is a drug treatment, sometimes taken in courses. The symptoms are fatigue, nausea, and decreased immunity. Light massage of short duration may be preferable, but negotiate with the client. Be aware that chemotherapy can cause thin skin. If you have any sort of infection yourself, do not massage but reschedule the treatment.

❻ Recent scar tissue is a local contraindication, and a potential site of infection. Do not massage if you have any infection yourself. Use supports as appropriate and negotiate comfortable positions with the client.

Breast cancer

Breast cancer can spread to the lymph nodes in the armpit, which are then surgically removed. This results in oedema in the arm on that side of the body. The client may be more comfortable with her arm elevated during the massage. Use light strokes only, towards the armpit, unless you are trained in manual lymphatic drainage.

If your client has had a mastectomy (removal of the breast, either whole or partial) be sensitive to her feelings about this, and take particular care with towel use.

HIV and AIDS

The Human Immuno-deficiency Virus (HIV) is transmitted in infected body fluids. Blood, seminal fluid and vaginal fluid contain high concentrations, and, for infection to occur, the virus must enter the bloodstream directly. Some symptoms of HIV infection include insomnia, night sweats, weight loss, diarrhoea, and skin disorders. With better combination drug treatments available, many HIV-positive people these days live ordinary lives.

Recommendations for massage

The virus is transmitted in body fluids, with high concentrations in semen, vaginal fluid and blood, and has a very short life outside the human body. There is no danger of contracting the virus if the normal rules of hygiene and avoiding open or weeping skin are observed. The benefits of massage for someone who is HIV-positive include relief from aches and pain, reduction in emotional stress, possible improvements in breathing, sleep patterns, and digestion, and possible improvements in the functioning of the immune system. If the person is fatigued, weak or unwell, use gentle massage. If medication is being injected, don't massage the site of an injection for an hour or so after administration. A person with AIDS has a seriously weakened immune system, so do not massage if you have an infection yourself. If someone has one of the opportunistic diseases, they may well be in hospital, and a doctor's advice should be sought.

Chapter 17
Endocrine disorders

Diabetes

Diabetes is the most common type of endocrine disorder that a massage therapist in general practice will encounter. The term refers to a group of diseases that involve metabolic or fluid disturbances in the body, which, if untreated, have serious long-term implications for health. Diabetes insipidus occurs when the posterior lobe of the pituitary gland, which produces the hormone ADH (antidiuretic hormone), is damaged. This usually occurs after a traumatic event, such as a skull fracture or brain surgery. Symptoms are excessive urination and thirst.

Diabetes mellitus is a disorder of the endocrine function of the pancreas gland. When the gland fails to produce enough insulin, blood sugar levels in the blood and urine rise. Symptoms include frequent urination, thirst, hunger, weight loss and tiredness. Long-term symptoms include susceptibility to infection, loss of sensation in peripheral nerves, damage to the eyes, and circulatory disorders. There are two common types. Type 1 has a sudden onset, and can occur in childhood. It is thought to be an auto-immune disorder. It carries more risks of long-term damage, and requires regular injections of insulin. Type 1 is more rare than Type 2, which develops slowly, later in life and affects more women than men. There is also a type of diabetes that occurs during pregnancy and disappears after the birth. Mild diabetes is controlled by medication, diet and exercise. A diabetic episode occurs if blood glucose gets too low (hypoglycaemia). The person becomes dizzy, hungry, irritable and weak.

Recommendations for massage

Gentle relaxation massage is beneficial for people with diabetes as long as they are healthy. Advise the medical practitioner that the client has sought massage. If the client takes regular medication, check that she has it with her in case of a diabetic episode. If the person injects insulin, avoid the injection site for an hour or so to avoid altering the rate of absorption of the drug. If there is loss of sensation in the peripheral nerves, be careful with pressure and when using manipulations or stretches. Long-term circulatory problems may cause thin skin in the peripheral areas of the body. Massage hands, feet and ankles gently, and take particular care over hygiene. Diabetics may experience other skin conditions, including itchy skin, spots or boils.

Seasonal affective disorder (SAD)

The pineal and pituitary glands in the brain regulate waking-sleeping rhythms and our responses to changes in the seasons. Imbalance between these two glands underlies seasonal affective disorder. Symptoms are weight gain, lethargy and depression, which vanish when the days get lighter and longer after winter.

Recommendations for massage

Relaxing massage may be helpful to relieve depression and tiredness.

THYROID DISORDERS

Underactive thyroid

Insufficient production of the hormone thyroxin by this gland means that the body cannot burn glucose to release energy. This results in weight gain, depression, fatigue and feeling cold. This condition is fairly common, occurring more often in women and in later life. If undiagnosed, people with underactive thyroids develop circulatory problems and fluid retention.

Recommendations for massage

Massage is beneficial if it can help someone with an underactive thyroid feel better about herself. If there are circulatory disorders, take appropriate precautions.

Overactive thyroid/Grave's disease

Overproduction of thyroxin causes the body to burn up fuel too quickly. Usually this is an auto-immune problem, in which case it is called Grave's disease. Symptoms are hyperactivity, difficulties sleeping and weight loss. It is treated with drugs or through the surgical removal of part of the gland. If the thyroid gland becomes enlarged as a result of too much or too little thyroxin, infection or inflammation, the swelling is called a goitre.

Recommendations for massage

Massage is beneficial if it helps the person to feel calmer. Avoid the neck area in a person with goitre.

Chapter 18
Digestive disorders

With all clients it is essential to follow the direction of the large intestine when doing firm massage on the abdomen, circling in a clockwise direction, so as not to risk pushing faecal material back into the small intestine. This may also assist the movement of faeces, and be helpful for relieving constipation.

Peristalsis in the digestive tract, and the secretion of digestive juices, are activities associated with parasympathetic nervous system activity. They occur when we are relaxed, and have energy available for the process, and cease in times of activity or stress, when energy is needed elsewhere in the body. Since many disorders of the digestive system are exacerbated by stress, relaxation massage of the whole body is helpful because it facilitates peristalsis and the secretion of digestive juices.

Conversely, massage of the abdomen is beneficial for someone with high levels of sympathetic nervous system arousal, because it helps the nervous system switch to parasympathetic.

DISORDERS OF THE DIGESTIVE TRACT

Constipation: recommendations for massage

If the cause is an abdominal obstruction, abdominal massage is a local contraindication. Otherwise, abdominal massage following the lines of the large intestine is recommended for constipation.

Nausea and vomiting

There are many factors that can cause nausea, including travel sickness, hormonal changes in early pregnancy, food poisoning, and bacterial infection. Nausea can lead to vomiting, which is one of the body's innate defence mechanisms for expelling harmful substances.

Recommendations for massage

Someone feeling nauseous probably wouldn't want a massage.

Gastro-enteritis

Nausea and vomiting, together with diarrhoea and raised temperature, are symptoms of gastro-enteritis, which means inflammation of any part of the digestive tract. The cause can be viral (the most common), bacterial or food intolerance.

Recommendations for massage

Acute gastro-enteritis is a contraindication to massage

because of the risk of infection to the practitioner and because the person probably wouldn't want one. This condition usually resolves in a few days. If the symptoms are longer term, they are probably associated with another digestive system disorder and relaxation massage, avoiding the abdomen, may be helpful for the reasons given above.

Indigestion or heartburn

Sometimes also called acid reflux, heartburn occurs when the sphincter at the end of the oesophagus malfunctions and acid from the stomach flows into the oesophagus.

Recommendations for massage

This condition can be worse after eating, so the client may be more comfortable to receive massage on an empty stomach. Lying flat may be uncomfortable, so consider propping the client into a semi-sitting position.

Ulcers

Ulcers of the stomach or duodenum cause burning pain in the upper abdomen and possibly bloating and gas. Stress, diet, smoking and alcohol may be contributing factors, although a common factor is also a bacterium that survives in the acidic environment of the stomach.

Recommendations for massage

Abdominal massage, except holds or gentle stroking, is contraindicated, but relaxation massage to restore autonomic functioning is beneficial.

DISORDERS OF THE LARGE INTESTINE

Ulcerative colitis

Ulcerative colitis refers to a condition where the mucous lining of the large intestine becomes inflamed and ulcers develop on the wall of the colon or rectum.

Crohn's disease

This is a progressive chronic inflammation of any part of the wall of the bowel. The symptoms are similar to ulcerative colitis, but it is a different condition.

Irritable bowel syndrome

This condition refers to a situation where the peristaltic waves in the bowel become irregular. However, there are no structural changes to the digestive tract as there are in conditions that have similar symptoms, such as ulcerative colitis or Crohn's disease. Diarrhoea alternates with constipation, the abdomen bloats and there are cramp-like pains.

Diverticulitis

This refers to little pouches that protrude outward on the wall of the large intestine, and can become inflected and painful. Constipation, diarrhoea, bloating and wind occur.

Recommendations for massage

Abdominal massage, except for holds and light stroking within the limits of tolerance of the client, is contraindicated for all these conditions. General relaxation massage to restore autonomic functioning is beneficial. Be sensitive to abdominal discomfort when the client lies on her front, and offer appropriate supports.

DISORDERS OF THE LIVER

Hepatitis

Hepatitis is inflammation of the liver. It can be caused by toxins, alcohol or prescribed drugs, or by a variety of infections. There are different kinds of infectious hepatitis, each having different modes of transmission and producing different symptoms with varying degrees of severity. Hepatitis A is short-lived with no lasting damage. Hepatitis B carries the risk of long-term complications, but the majority of hepatitis C carriers do not develop chronic infection. The virus is carried in faeces and body fluids, and can survive outside the body. Symptoms of hepatitis are lethargy, nausea, weakness, temperature and possibly jaundice, which causes yellowish skin and eyes, from the excess of the pigment bilirubin in the blood. Not everyone who has hepatitis has symptoms, which means a person may have the disease without knowing.

Recommendations for massage

Hepatitis is a contraindication to massage while it is

infectious. This stage varies from type to type, so it is advisable to consult with the medical practitioner first about the advisability of massage. Avoid abdominal massage, particularly in the area of the liver, on someone with chronic hepatitis, and avoid techniques that stimulate the circulation and could put pressure on a weakened liver. Adapt the massage and the duration of the treatment to the general vitality of the person. Take particular care with usual hygiene precautions, and do not massage if you yourself have an infectious disease, because a hepatitis sufferer's immune system is compromised. There is no reason not to massage a person who has recovered from hepatitis normally.

Cirrhosis

Cirrhosis of the liver occurs when healthy liver cells die and are replaced with fatty fibrous tissues, causing liver malfunction and possibly death. There are many possible causes, including hepatitis and alcoholism. It may be symptomless initially, and then leads to vomiting and weight loss, and finally to a range of serious disruptions to many other body systems.

Recommendations for massage

If the cirrhosis is connected to hepatitis, do not massage during the acute stage and get medical advice. Avoid abdominal massage, circulatory massage, and, if there is oedema in the legs, avoid draining techniques on the legs.

Gall stones

These are hard little deposits of cholesterol or bilirubin in the gallbladder. A person with gall stones may not be aware of their existence, but when the stones try to pass down the bile duct they cause severe pain.

Recommendations for massage

Do not massage during an attack, although the person would be too ill to want a massage. At other times, massage should be fine, but avoid deep work in the area of the liver.

HERNIAS

Hernias develop when there is a weakness in the muscles around the abdominal cavity, which allows an organ, or part of it, to protrude. Hernias can be pushed back (don't attempt to do this!) and disappear when the person lies down.

Hiatus hernia

This refers to a condition where part of the stomach protrudes through the diaphragm into the thorax, and gastric juices may flow into the oesophagus, causing acid reflux. It is more common in older people.

Inguinal hernia

The place where the testis and sperm duct descend through the abdominal wall in a young boy remains a potential weak spot where the intestines or bladder can protrude later in life.

Abdominal hernia

Hernias can arise where the muscle of the abdominal wall has been cut through for major surgery.

Femoral hernia

Another site of weakness is the place where the femoral artery passes through, in the groin.

Recommendations for massage

Whatever the cause, hernias are a local contraindication to massage. A person with a hiatus hernia will be more comfortable sitting than lying, and should be massaged with the upper body raised.

Chapter 19
Female reproductive processes

As well as the common disorders and medical conditions relating to the reproductive system that may crop up in an everyday massage practice, there are also considerations relating to normal processes of the female reproductive system for the massage therapist to be aware of.

Menstruation: recommendations for massage

During the two weeks before menstruation many women experience some of the signs of pre-menstrual syndrome (PMS), such as fluid retention, sore breasts, irritability, sugar cravings, fatigue, or headaches. Soothing massage may be helpful. Lymphatic drainage techniques may ease congestion. During a period some women experience abdominal cramps, or sensitivity in the abdomen, lower back or thighs. Massage of these areas may be helpful or completely unwanted. Negotiation is important, and proper use of supports is needed for sore breasts or abdomens. Avoid deep abdominal massage. Sensitivity is also needed for women who bleed very heavily and need to wear heavy feminine protection, or to change during a treatment.

Constipation is not uncommon before a period. There is some evidence that abdominal massage may help.

Pregnancy: recommendations for massage

During the first three months of pregnancy there is a high risk of miscarriage, and all massage on the abdomen is contraindicated, for practitioner protection. After that stage, deep abdominal massage continues to be contraindicated throughout pregnancy and for several weeks after birth.

Positioning and supports are important. During the initial stages, a women can receive massage in the usual positions, but in the later stages she cannot lie on her stomach, and needs to lie on her side, or to be supported in a sitting position. When lying on her back, she needs good support under her knees. Avoid the supine position for too long, because of the pressure of the foetus on the abdominal blood vessels. Hormonal changes loosen all ligaments and tendons in the body, so avoid, or take particular care with, joint manipulations and stretches.

Menopause: recommendations for massage

This stage involves adjustment on an emotional as well as physical level, and relaxing massage may help with the stresses of this transition. The one symptom consistently associated with menopause is hot flushes. Be aware that these sudden changes in body temperature may require a client to have different layers of coverings available during a treatment.

Chapter 20
Reproductive system disorders

DISORDERS OF THE FEMALE REPRODUCTIVE SYSTEM

Fibroids

Fibroids are slow-growing, benign tumours of the uterus wall. They are rarely painful but can cause heavy periods and a dragging sensation in the abdomen. Fibroids often shrink after menopause.

Recommendations for massage

Deep abdominal massage is contraindicated for large fibroids.

Endometriosis

This means the presence of tissue from the inside of the uterus growing in other places in the body, usually in the abdominal cavity. These patches of endometrial tissue swell and break down in line with the menstrual cycle. Periods may be painful, and there may be abdominal tenderness and other symptoms. It is a long-term condition, which may cause infertility.

Recommendations for massage

Deep abdominal massage is contraindicated. Relaxation massage is beneficial to ameliorate the anxiety and stress caused by living with the condition.

Pelvic inflammatory disease

Pelvic inflammatory disease is the infection of the uterus and ovaries, with pain, tenderness in the abdomen and a high temperature.

Recommendations for massage

Deep abdominal massage is contraindicated. The client may be more comfortable with her knees bent.

Prolapse

Women who have had children may find that the pelvic floor muscles lose their elasticity, and their ability to support the organs in the lower abdomen, particularly after the menopause. A prolapse involves the uterus or vagina descending from its normal position and possibly protruding outside the body.

Recommendations for massage

Abdominal massage is contraindicated, and avoid hip joint

manipulations. Take care to offer appropriate supports when the client is lying on her front.

MALE REPRODUCTIVE DISORDERS

Prostate cancer

This form of cancer is common in elderly men. Symptoms vary according to the stage of disease and the treatment used.

Recommendations for massage

See the general recommendations for cancer and massage. Prostate cancer is not a contraindication to massage, but note that there can be a need to urinate more frequently. Relaxation massage can help reduce associated anxiety.

Chapter 21
Sexually transmitted diseases

There is an Act of Parliament from 1917 prohibiting the use of complementary therapies to treat syphilis, gonorrhoea or soft chancre (genital sores). Massage does not claim to treat, in the sense of diagnose and cure, medical conditions, but practitioners should be aware of this law.

Syphilis

Syphilis is a bacterial infection that is sexually transmitted. The initial symptoms are fluid-filled painless lesions. Untreated, the disease affects many systems, and it used to be fatal.

Recommendations for massage

Syphilitic lesions contain highly infectious material, so, in this stage of the disease, massage is totally contraindicated. Once the lesions are treated, seek medical advice about the advisability of massage and observe contraindications for other symptoms.

Gonorrhoea

This is a bacterial condition transmitted only by sexual contact, so it is of no risk to the practitioner. Massage can be given as normal.

Genital herpes

The same herpes simplex virus that causes cold sores on the mouth causes genital herpes. Once this virus has entered the body it lies dormant. Attacks are usually precipitated by stress. There is prickling in the area, leading to eruptions of painful sores that burst and disappear after a week or so.

Recommendations for massage

During an attack, the client may prefer to keep his/her underwear on. The virus is highly infectious and remains alive outside the host body for some hours, so be particularly careful with the usual hygiene precautions. Many sufferers of genital herpes are very ashamed of the condition and feel dirty during an attack. Be sensitive to this.

Genital infestations

Pubic lice and scabies are highly infectious and can be transmitted through contact with infected linen.

Recommendations for massage

Genital infestations are a total contraindication to massage until cleared up.

Chapter 22
Massage and sexuality

The old connection between massage and massage parlour is diminishing, as the massage therapy profession develops rigorous standards for training and registration of its practitioners, and research into the effectiveness of massage techniques provides scientific credibility. Unfortunately, however, there are still some individuals who book a massage treatment expecting sexual services, and therapists need to know how to deal with this.

Both non-sexual massage and sexual contact involve touch, and the nature of that touch can be very similar, even though the context (treatment room rather than bedroom) and the intention of the giver (massage therapist rather than lover) are different, a body could be forgiven for interpreting long, slow effleurage strokes as sexual caresses, even when the mind knows full well that this is not the intention.

On occasion, sexual arousal can occur innocently during massage, more obviously in men, who are usually extremely embarrassed by an unwanted erection.

What to do when a man gets an erection during a massage

If the client seems uncomfortable or embarrassed, try one of the following. Ignore the erection and carry on with the massage. Or you could say something like: "I notice you've got an erection. Don't worry, it happens. It will go away."

Avoid potentially arousing areas, such as the inside thighs or buttocks. If you sense that the man is enjoying being sexually aroused, or if he asks you to touch his penis, be clear that you are not performing sexual services and terminate the treatment.

Chapter 23
Urinary system disorders

Massage is only contraindicated for urinary disorders if there is localised pain, fever or the person is very unwell. Avoiding the abdomen is a sensible precaution, particularly if the client needs to urinate often. Be sensitive to potential embarrassment or shame associated with these conditions, especially incontinence. Allow time for visits to the bathroom during the treatment.

URINARY TRACT INFECTIONS

These common infections cause burning pain when urinating, often caused by bacterial infection from the digestive tract.

Cystitis

Cystitis is inflammation of the ureters and/or bladder. The symptoms are pain and an urgent, frequent need to urinate. All urinary tract infections are more common in women because of the relative shortness of the ureter, which means that the rest of the urinary tract is more exposed to the external environment than in men.

Recommendations for massage

Avoid abdominal massage. Bear in mind that the client may need to visit the toilet during the treatment. Encourage fluid intake.

Kidney stones

These are small hard deposits found in the kidneys, more often in men. Lack of fluid can be a causative factor, so they are more commonly diagnosed in hot weather. Most stones are too small to be a problem and are passed through the ureters to the bladder and out of the body in urine. Larger ones can cause severe pain, called renal colic, when they are passing down the ureters.

Recommendations for massage

There is no reason not to massage someone with a history of kidney stones, unless he is suffering from renal colic, in which case massage is contraindicated and he probably would be too ill to want one anyway.

Gout

If the kidneys fail to remove uric acid (a metabolic waste product), the build-up in the blood forms crystals that settle in the joints, causing a form of arthritis. The most commonly affected joints are in the feet, particularly the big toe. An attack is very sudden and very painful. The affected joint becomes red, shiny and extremely painful.

Recommendations for massage

Massage is contraindicated in the acute stage, and wouldn't be wanted. Gouty joints are a local contraindication although massage of surrounding areas can help circulation.

Incontinence

More common in the elderly and in women who have had children, incontinence is involuntary urination. Stress incontinence, release of small amounts of urine, can occur when a person laughs or undertakes strenuous activity. In severe cases of incontinence a catheter may be fitted.

Recommendations for massage

Be sensitive and try to put the client at ease. If a catheter is worn, negotiate comfort and use of supports. If the client wears incontinence pads, ensure the area is respectfully covered by a towel during the treatment. Allow more time for dressing and undressing and trips to the bathroom. Avoid abdominal massage.

Renal failure

Renal failure means that the kidneys have stopped functioning. It can be acute or chronic, developing over a number of years. It is a condition that affects nearly all the systems of the body. Treatment is with dialysis on a kidney machine.

Recommendations for massage

Don't massage during the acute stage and then consult with the medical practitioner first about the advisability of massage. Use light massage only to avoid pressure on the circulatory system, and keep treatments short. If oedema is present, treat as a local contraindication. Be aware of the possibility of thin skin and fragile bones. If the client is on dialysis, avoid the site of connection.

References

British National Formulary
British Medical Association and the Royal Pharmaceutical Society of Great Britain
Copies from BMJ bookshop, PO Box 295, London WC1H 9TE.
www.BNF.org

Anatomy, Physiology and Pathology for the Massage Therapist
Su Fox and Darien Pritchard
2001 Corpus Publishing

Report on Contraindications in Massage
The General Council of Massage Therapy, Training and Education section
2004 GCMT

Black's Medical Dictionary
Gordon MacPherson (ed.)
2002 A & C Black

Healthy Living
PPP healthcare
2001 PPP healthcare

Massage Therapy and Medications
Randal S. Persad
2002 Curties-Overzet Publications Inc.

Pathology A to Z – a handbook for massage therapists
Kalyani Premkuma
1996 VanPub Books

The Body Remembers – The psychophysiology of trauma and trauma treatment
Babette Rothschild
2000 W.W. Norton and Co.

Massage Therapy: Principles and Practice
Susan Salvo
1999, W.B. Saunders Co. New York

The British Medical Association Complete Family Health Encyclopaedia
Dr. Tony Smith (ed.)
1990 Dorling Kindersley

The Penguin Medical Encyclopaedia
Peter Wingate and Richard Wingate
1996 Penguin Books

A Massage Therapist's Guide to Pathology
Ruth Werner
2002 Lippincott Williams and Wilkins

Index

A
Abdominal hernia 141
Acne vulgaris 60
Acupuncture 6
Age spots 67
AIDS 4, 15, 19, 69, 123, 128-129
Allergies 14, 39, 65, 123-124
Alzheimer's disease 114
Anaemia 39, 72-73
Analgesics 16, 20, 26
Anaphylactic shock 125
Anatomy 7
Angiogram 30
Ankylosing spondylitis 50
Antibiotics 16, 26, 36, 87
Anticoagulants 24, 25
Antidepressants 11, 16, 23
Antihistamines 25
Anxiety 23-24, 81, 109, 117, 120-121, 146
Arteriogram 30
Arteriosclerosis 71, 75, 80
Arthritis 14, 20-21, 31, 38-39, 47-50, 95, 123, 152
Asthma 8, 21, 26, 65, 88, 124
Athlete's foot 5, 34, 63

B
Bedsores 67
Bell's palsy 96-97
Beta blockers 24
Blisters 61, 66-67, 97
Blood cancer 73
Boils 60-61, 131
Bone-density scan 51
Breast cancer 29, 128
British Medical Association 17
British National Formulary 9, 17
Bronchitis 14, 32, 83-84, 86-87
Bronchodilators 25, 26
Bruising 16, 34, 43, 66
Bursitis 46

C
Cancer 14-15, 19, 23, 31, 39, 69, 73, 76, 89, 123, 126-127
Cancer, blood 73
Cancer, breast 29, 128
Cancer, colon 126
Cancer, lung 89, 126
Cancer, pancreas 126
Cancer, prostate 19, 126, 146
Cancer, skin 68-69
Cancer, uterus 126
Candida 63
Carbuncles 60, 131
Cardiovascular conditions 15, 20, 24, 71-90
Carpal tunnel syndrome 45, 95
Cellulitis 66
Cerebral palsy 105
Cerebrovascular accident 99
Chemical dependency 119-120
Chiropractor 11, 45, 101
Chronic fatigue syndrome 106, 125
Cirrhosis 15, 139
Colds 14, 33, 35, 74, 83-85
Colon cancer 126
Common allergies 14, 39, 65, 123
Communication difficulty 103, 105, 112-116
Complementary therapy 5-6, 9-10
Constipation 14, 134-135, 137, 143
Corticosteroids 21

Coughs 14, 26, 84, 86-87, 90
Counselling 6, 122
Cramp 13, 54-55, 81, 91, 137
Crohn's disease 14, 137
Crying 121
CT scan 28
CVA 99
Cystitis 151

D
Decongestants 26
Deep tissue massage 16, 20, 21, 27
Deep vein thrombosis 33, 71, 79
Dementia 114-115
Depression 23, 121, 132
Dermatitis 64-65
DEXA scan 28
Diabetes 14, 80, 94-95, 109, 130-131
Diarrhoea 14, 129, 135-136
Diuretics 24, 25
Diverticulitis 137
Doctor 6, 9-15, 17-18, 24-25, 31, 34, 44, 50, 58, 71-72, 76, 81-82, 100, 129
Drowsiness 25, 26
Drugs 16-24, 26, 120, 128-129, 131, 133, 138
Dyslexia 113

E
Eating disorders 119
ECG 30, 31
Eczema 58-60, 64-65, 124
EEG 31
Emotional vulnerability 113, 117-122
Emphysema 14, 87
Endocrine disorders 14, 130-133
Endometriosis 144
Endoscopy 29
Epilepsy 98, 114
ESR 31

F
Femoral hernia 141
Fibroids 144

Fibromyalgia 14, 55
Fibromyositis 55
Fibrosis 39, 55
Fibrositis 55
Fractures 14, 23, 29, 34, 40-41
Friction strokes 21, 44, 47, 68, 70, 95, 102
Frozen shoulder 46

G
Gallstones 14, 139-140
Gastro-enteritis 135
Genital herpes 61-62, 148
Genital infestations 148
Gonorrhoea 147-148
Gout 153-154
Grave's disease 132-133

H
Haemophilia 39, 74
Hay fever 14, 65, 124
Headaches 42, 98, 101
Head lice 64
Hearing impairment 14, 110
Heart attack 33, 71, 80-82
Heartburn 136
Heart failure 25, 76, 82
Hepatitis 15, 138-139
Hernia 140-141
Hernia, abdominal 141
Hernia, femoral 141
Hernia, hiatus 140-141
Hernia, inguinal 140
Herniated disc 44-45, 96, 101
Herpes simplex 61-62, 148
Herpes zoster 97
Hiatus hernia 140-141
Hickman line 19
HIV 15, 19, 90, 123, 128-129
Homoeopathy 6
Hygiene 21, 37, 59, 61-63, 85, 129, 131, 139, 148
Hypertension 74-75
Hypotension 75

I

IBS 14
Impetigo 59, 61
Implants 19
Incontinence 108, 151, 153
Indigestion 136
Infection 14, 16, 21, 26, 33-37, 57-62, 66, 74, 83-84, 86-87, 89-90, 93-94, 128-130, 135-136, 138, 145, 147, 151
Inflammation 19-21, 29, 34, 46-47, 49-50, 60, 65, 76, 83, 85-87, 89, 94, 97, 100, 123-124, 133, 135, 137-138, 151
Influenza 85, 66, 106
Inguinal hernia 140
Injection 18-20, 28, 129, 131
Irritable bowel syndrome 14

J/K

Jet lag 14
Kidney stones 14, 153
Kyphosis 53

L

Laryngitis 86
Learning impairment 113-114
Leukaemia 73
Liver spots 67
Lordosis 53
Lung cancer 89, 126

M

Malpractice 12, 13
Mammogram 29
Meningitis 94, 100-101
Menopause 14, 51, 143-145
Menstruation 14, 91, 142, 144
Migraine 98
Miscarriage 14, 143
MRI scan 27, 29
MRSA 36-37
Multiple sclerosis 94, 104, 115, 123
Muscle relaxants 22, 23
Muscle spasm 22, 45, 55, 57, 101
Muscular dystrophy 14, 56
Myasthenia gravis 56-57, 123
Myocardial infarction 81

N

Naturopathy 6
Nausea 81, 128, 135, 138
Nervous system disorders 14, 93-105, 112
Neuralgia 94, 97
Neuritis 94
Neuropathy 94
Nits 65
NSAIDs 20-21

O

Oedema 25, 70, 76, 82, 128, 139, 154
Opiates 22
Osteoarthritis 20, 38, 48-49
Osteomalacia 52
Osteoporosis 14, 28, 38, 50-52
Overactive thyroid 132-133

P

Pacemaker 82
Pancreatic cancer 126
Panic attacks 120-121
Parkinson's disease 94, 103
Pathology 5-8
Pelvic inflammatory disease 145
Percussion techniques 21, 44, 70, 86
Pleurisy 89
Pneumonia 14, 59, 83-84, 87
Polarity therapy 6
Poliomyelitis 94, 103, 106
Post-traumatic stress 117-119
Pregnancy 14, 32, 45, 68, 76, 78-79, 131, 135, 143
Pressure sores 67
Prolapse 145
Prostate cancer 19, 146
Psoriasis 21, 48, 65
Psychotherapy 6, 122
Pulmonary TB 15, 83, 90

Q/R

Raynaud's disease 77
Relaxation 6-7, 24, 45, 48-49, 87-89, 92, 97, 109, 111, 114, 116, 119, 121, 126, 131, 134-136, 145-146
Renal failure 152-153
Repetitive strain injury 21, 38, 45, 95, 103
Rheumatism 47
Rheumatoid arthritis 20-21, 39, 49, 95, 123
Rickets 52
Ringworm 62-63
Royal Pharmaceutical Society 17

S

Seasonal affective disorder 131-132
Scabies 63-64, 148
Sciatica 95, 101
Scoliosis 53
Sexually transmitted disorders 61, 147-150
Shiatsu 6
Shingles 97
Side effects 16-17, 23-24, 39
Sinusitis 14, 85
Skin, cancer 68-69
Skin, conditions and disorders 14, 18, 21, 58-70, 124, 131
Skin, tags 68
Skin, thin 21, 66, 68-70, 76, 89, 102, 104, 119, 128, 131, 154
Slipped disc 44-45, 96, 101
Spina bifida 94, 102-103
Spinal cord 44, 91-92, 94, 96, 100-105
Spinal curvature 53-54
Sport injuries 7, 40, 42-44, 80
Sprains 13, 42-43, 91
Stomach ulcers 136
Strains 14, 21, 26, 36, 42-47, 55, 95
Stress 7, 32, 49, 61, 69, 71, 75, 81, 89, 98, 103, 109, 111, 117-119, 121, 127, 129, 134, 136, 143, 145, 148, 153

Stretch marks 68
Stroke 12, 33, 80, 94, 99-100, 115
Superbugs 36
Syphilis 147

T

TB 15, 83, 90
Tendinitis 46-47
Thin skin 21, 66, 68-70, 76, 89, 102, 104, 119, 128, 131, 154
Thrombophlebitis 78-79
Thrombosis 33, 71, 78-79, 99
Thrush 63
Thyroid disorders 14, 31, 132-133
TIA 100
Tinnitus 111
Tranquillisers 23, 37-38, 40, 74, 91, 93, 117-119, 130
Transient ischaemic attack 100
Trauma 35
Trigeminal neuralgia 97
Tuberculosis 90

U

Ulcerative colitis 137
Ulcers 136-137
Ultrasound 29
Underactive thyroid 132
Urinary tract infections 151
Uterus cancer

V

Varicose veins 65, 70, 77-78
Vasodilators 24-25
Verrucas 62
Visual impairment 109
Vitiligo 67, 123
Vomiting 119, 135, 139

W/X/Y/Z

Warts 62
X-ray 27-30